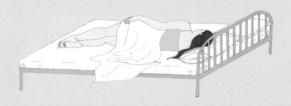

HOW TO USE THIS JOURNAL

Decoding your dreams can offer you incredible insight into yourself and your life. Every night, your dreaming mind is gently and subtly counseling, guiding, and inspiring you. Unfortunately, many of us don't make dream recall and interpretation a daily ritual and miss out on an incredible opportunity for personal growth.

Most modern dream experts believe that your dreams act like an internal therapist. The messages they send you have the potential to heal and transform your life. Humans throughout history and across cultures have understood the potential of dreams to inform and offer insight into our waking lives. According to the Talmud, "a dream which is not interpreted is like a letter which is not read."

If you want to interpret your dreams and benefit from the empowering wisdom of your night vision, the first crucial step is to actually remember them. Even if you are one of those people who feels they never dream, you do. You just need to train yourself to recall the details. Making a habit of writing in your dream journal every day will help program your mind for dream recall, as will these sleep hygiene tips and dream recall steps.

BEFORE BED

- Place this dream journal beside your bed with a pen or pencil.

- Aim to keep your bedroom as dark and as noiseproof as possible.
  A temperature of around 60–65°F (16–18°C) is considered optimum
  for sleep.

- Avoid exercise, alcohol, and caffeine before bed.

- Avoid looking at screens for at least an hour before you go to bed.

- Keep to regular sleeping and waking times every day. If you can wake
  up without an alarm clock, all the better, as dream recall improves when
  waking naturally.

- If you have the *Dream Decoder* cards, you may want to select one at random
  and meditate on it gently for a few minutes before going to bed. Hold that
  image in mind as you let go of your thoughts and settle down to sleep.

ON WAKING

Make writing down your dreams the very first part of your morning ritual,
otherwise your dream memories will quickly melt away. Don't be tempted to
get up, stretch, have a shower, brush your teeth, or check your phone before
using this journal. Getting out of bed and focusing on the day ahead will
distract you from dream recall.

If you wake with a great deal of detail from your dream in mind, turn straight
to the space reserved for bigger dreams, the ones at the start of the journal
that go over two pages. If you remember just the odd detail, use one of the
small, half-page sections toward the back. Turn to the relevant page and pour
out whatever you can recall. If details start flooding back to you as you write,
don't worry about running out of space—just continue down the page and
over to the next if need be, ignoring the existing headings. At this stage, don't
try to interpret your dream; simply write down anything and everything you
can remember.

Be sure to write in the present tense to keep the dreams as fresh and alive
as possible. Don't try to make your dream tell a story or make sense—just
write down any images, impressions, or insights that arise (note down

specific sounds, people, symbols, animals, colors, places, scenes, and whatever else has stuck with you). Most importantly, pay attention to the feelings you experienced during the dream, as they will prove crucial for your interpretation.

When you have written down all you can remember and identified the dominant emotion, have a go at drawing something from your dream. It doesn't need to be a work of art—just draw whatever your dream inspires. Don't forget to make a note of the date and time.

Leave the interpretation section blank for now: it's best to give yourself some distance from a dream rather than interpreting it immediately. Put the journal away, get on with your day, and then reflect on it later, perhaps in the evening.

KEEP UP WITH YOUR DREAM JOURNAL

Aim to write in your dream journal every day for at least four weeks—research suggests this is the minimum time it takes for a new habit or daily ritual to become second nature. When you have a few weeks of dreams recorded, glance through them again, as hindsight can be a great teacher. You may well find that your dreaming past is a treasure trove of inspiration or insight.

IS IT ALL A DREAM?

On very rare occasions you may become aware that you are dreaming while you are still dreaming—this is called lucid dreaming. It's wildly exciting because in a lucid dream you can take charge of the story and do or be whatever you want. To increase your chances of lucid dreaming, get into the habit of asking yourself if you are awake or dreaming whenever you perform a routine action during the day, such as checking the time. The idea is that if you check the time in your dream, you will automatically ask yourself the same question and will realize in your dream that you are asleep.

Related to lucid dreaming is false awakening, a phenomenon in which you are still asleep but dream of having awoken. You may get out of bed, get dressed, eat breakfast, and otherwise go about your daily routine in the belief that you are awake before actually waking up. Unlike lucid dreaming, you will not be aware that you are sleeping, though false awakening may occur immediately before or after a lucid dream.

FALLING

SEE P. 132 FOR THIS DREAM'S INTERPRETATION

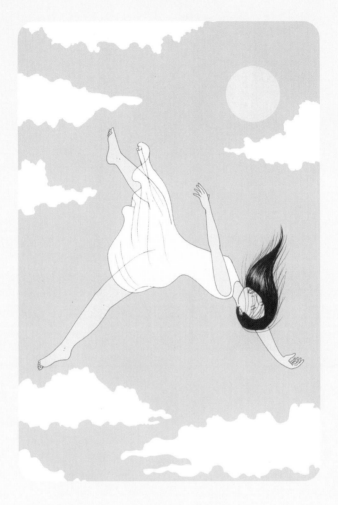

What does falling while dreaming feel like?

....
....
....
....
....
....

NUDITY

SEE P. 133 FOR THIS DREAM'S INTERPRETATION

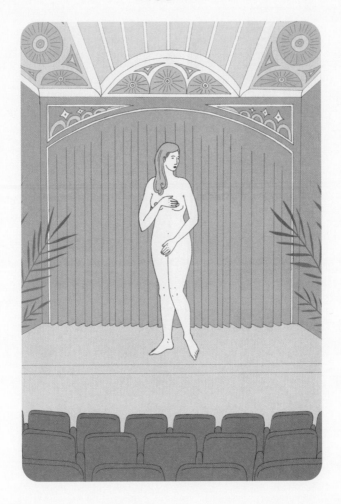

How have you experienced nudity in a dream?

....
....
....
....
....
....

BEING UNPREPARED

SEE P. 131 FOR THIS DREAM'S INTERPRETATION

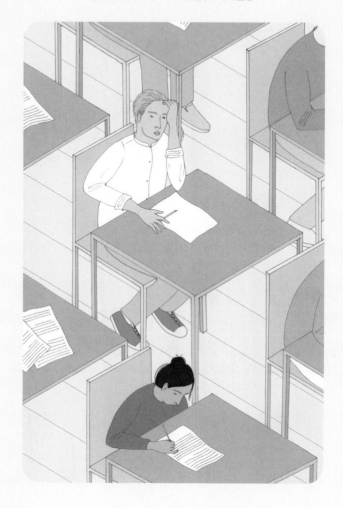

Does this sound familiar to you?

UNABLE TO FIND A BATHROOM

SEE P. 135 FOR THIS DREAM'S INTERPRETATION

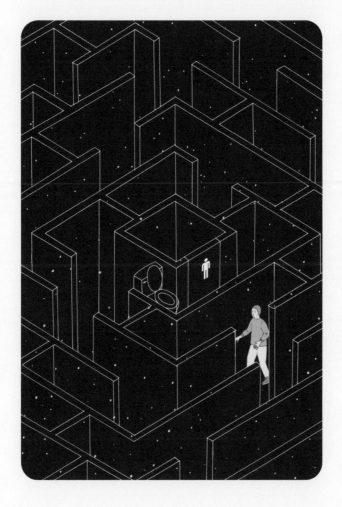

How does this dream make you feel?

BEING CHASED

SEE P. 137 FOR THIS DREAM'S INTERPRETATION

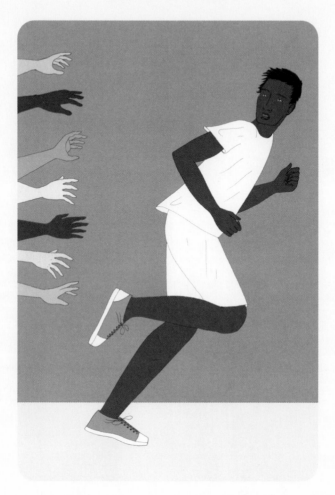

How does it feel to be chased in a dream?

TEETH FALLING OUT

SEE P. 135 FOR THIS DREAM'S INTERPRETATION

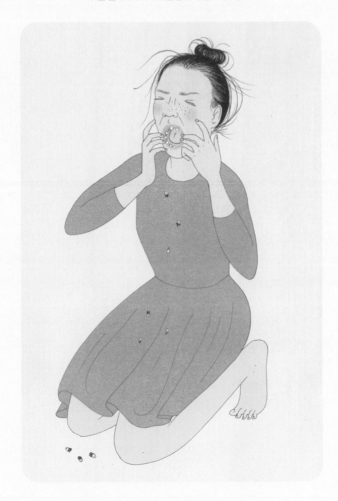

Have you ever dreamed about this?

Title: _____ Date/Time: _____ Location: _____

How did it make you feel?

☐ Excited   ☐ Overwhelmed   ☐ Anxious
☐ Happy   ☐ Confused   ☐ Scared
☐ Emotional   ☐ Worried   ☐ Vulnerable
☐ Relaxed   ☐ Frustrated   ☐ ....

Are there any recurring themes?

_____
_____
_____
_____
_____

How would you draw your dream?

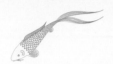

How would you interpret this dream?

Any related memories from the day before?

_____

_____

_____

_____

What was the moon phase?

Title: _____ Date/Time: _____ Location: _____

How did it make you feel?

☐ Excited ☐ Overwhelmed ☐ Anxious
☐ Happy   ☐ Confused   ☐ Scared
☐ Emotional ☐ Worried   ☐ Vulnerable
☐ Relaxed ☐ Frustrated   ☐ ....

Are there any recurring themes?

_____
_____
_____
_____
_____

How would you draw your dream?

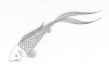

How would you interpret this dream?

Any related memories from the day before?

_____

_____

_____

_____

What was the moon phase?

Title: _____ Date/Time: _____ Location: _____

How did it make you feel?

Are there any recurring themes?

☐ Excited   ☐ Overwhelmed   ☐ Anxious

☐ Happy   ☐ Confused   ☐ Scared

☐ Emotional   ☐ Worried   ☐ Vulnerable

☐ Relaxed   ☐ Frustrated   ☐ ....

_____
_____
_____
_____
_____

How would you draw your dream?

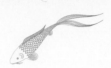

How would you interpret this dream?

Any related memories from the day before?

What was the moon phase?

Title: _____ Date/Time: _____ Location: _____

How did it make you feel?

Are there any recurring themes?

	Excited		Overwhelmed		Anxious
	Happy		Confused		Scared
	Emotional		Worried		Vulnerable
	Relaxed		Frustrated		....

_____
_____
_____
_____
_____

How would you draw your dream?

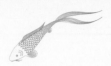

How would you interpret this dream?

Any related memories from the day before?

_____

_____

_____

_____

_____

What was the moon phase?

Title: _____ Date/Time: _____ Location: _____

How did it make you feel?

☐ Excited ☐ Overwhelmed ☐ Anxious
☐ Happy ☐ Confused ☐ Scared
☐ Emotional ☐ Worried ☐ Vulnerable
☐ Relaxed ☐ Frustrated ☐ ....

Are there any recurring themes?

_____
_____
_____
_____
_____

How would you draw your dream?

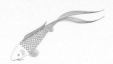

How would you interpret this dream?

Any related memories from the day before?

What was the moon phase?

Title: _____ Date/Time: _____ Location: _____

How did it make you feel?

☐ Excited   ☐ Overwhelmed   ☐ Anxious
☐ Happy   ☐ Confused   ☐ Scared
☐ Emotional ☐ Worried   ☐ Vulnerable
☐ Relaxed   ☐ Frustrated   ☐ ....

Are there any recurring themes?

_____
_____
_____
_____
_____

How would you draw your dream?

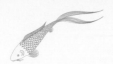

How would you interpret this dream?

Any related memories from the day before?

What was the moon phase?

Title: _____ Date/Time: _____ Location: _____

How did it make you feel?

- [ ] Excited
- [ ] Happy
- [ ] Emotional
- [ ] Relaxed

- [ ] Overwhelmed
- [ ] Confused
- [ ] Worried
- [ ] Frustrated

- [ ] Anxious
- [ ] Scared
- [ ] Vulnerable
- [ ] ....

Are there any recurring themes?

_____
_____
_____
_____
_____

How would you draw your dream?

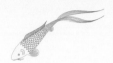

How would you interpret this dream?

Any related memories from the day before?

_____

_____

_____

_____

_____

What was the moon phase?

Title: _____ Date/Time: _____ Location: _____

How did it make you feel?

☐ Excited   ☐ Overwhelmed   ☐ Anxious
☐ Happy   ☐ Confused   ☐ Scared
☐ Emotional   ☐ Worried   ☐ Vulnerable
☐ Relaxed   ☐ Frustrated   ☐ ....

Are there any recurring themes?

_____
_____
_____
_____
_____

How would you draw your dream?

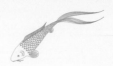

How would you interpret this dream?

Any related memories from the day before?

What was the moon phase?

Title: _____ Date/Time: _____ Location: _____

How did it make you feel?

Are there any recurring themes?

- [ ] Excited
- [ ] Happy
- [ ] Emotional
- [ ] Relaxed
- [ ] Overwhelmed
- [ ] Confused
- [ ] Worried
- [ ] Frustrated
- [ ] Anxious
- [ ] Scared
- [ ] Vulnerable
- [ ] ....

_____
_____
_____
_____
_____

How would you draw your dream?

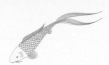

How would you interpret this dream?

Any related memories from the day before?

What was the moon phase?

Title: _____ Date/Time: _____ Location: _____

How did it make you feel?

☐ Excited   ☐ Overwhelmed   ☐ Anxious

☐ Happy   ☐ Confused   ☐ Scared

☐ Emotional   ☐ Worried   ☐ Vulnerable

☐ Relaxed   ☐ Frustrated   ☐ ....

Are there any recurring themes?

_____
_____
_____
_____
_____

How would you draw your dream?

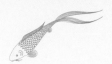

How would you interpret this dream?

Any related memories from the day before?

_____

_____

_____

_____

_____

What was the moon phase?

Title: _____ Date/Time: _____ Location: _____

How did it make you feel?

☐ Excited	☐ Overwhelmed	☐ Anxious	
☐ Happy	☐ Confused	☐ Scared	
☐ Emotional	☐ Worried	☐ Vulnerable	
☐ Relaxed	☐ Frustrated	☐	

Are there any recurring themes?

_____
_____
_____
_____
_____

How would you draw your dream?

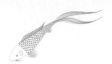

How would you interpret this dream?

Any related memories from the day before?

What was the moon phase?

Title: _____ Date/Time: _____ Location: _____

How did it make you feel?

Are there any recurring themes?

☐	Excited	☐	Overwhelmed	☐	Anxious
☐	Happy	☐	Confused	☐	Scared
☐	Emotional	☐	Worried	☐	Vulnerable
☐	Relaxed	☐	Frustrated	☐	....

_____
_____
_____
_____
_____

How would you draw your dream?

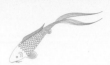

How would you interpret this dream?

Any related memories from the day before?

What was the moon phase?

Title: _____ Date/Time: _____ Location: _____

How did it make you feel?

Are there any recurring themes?

- [ ] Excited
- [ ] Happy
- [ ] Emotional
- [ ] Relaxed

- [ ] Overwhelmed
- [ ] Confused
- [ ] Worried
- [ ] Frustrated

- [ ] Anxious
- [ ] Scared
- [ ] Vulnerable
- [ ] ....

_____
_____
_____
_____
_____

How would you draw your dream?

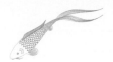

How would you interpret this dream?

Any related memories from the day before?

What was the moon phase?

Title: _____ Date/Time: _____ Location: _____

How did it make you feel?

☐ Excited ☐ Overwhelmed ☐ Anxious
☐ Happy ☐ Confused ☐ Scared
☐ Emotional ☐ Worried ☐ Vulnerable
☐ Relaxed ☐ Frustrated ☐ ....

Are there any recurring themes?

_____
_____
_____
_____
_____

How would you draw your dream?

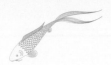

How would you interpret this dream?

Any related memories from the day before?

What was the moon phase?

Title: _____ Date/Time: _____ Location: _____

How did it make you feel?

Are there any recurring themes?

- [ ] Excited
- [ ] Happy
- [ ] Emotional
- [ ] Relaxed

- [ ] Overwhelmed
- [ ] Confused
- [ ] Worried
- [ ] Frustrated

- [ ] Anxious
- [ ] Scared
- [ ] Vulnerable
- [ ] ....

_____
_____
_____
_____
_____

How would you draw your dream?

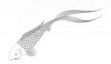

How would you interpret this dream?

Any related memories from the day before?

_____

_____

_____

_____

_____

What was the moon phase?

Title: _____ Date/Time: _____ Location: _____

How did it make you feel?

☐ Excited   ☐ Overwhelmed   ☐ Anxious
☐ Happy   ☐ Confused   ☐ Scared
☐ Emotional ☐ Worried   ☐ Vulnerable
☐ Relaxed   ☐ Frustrated   ☐ ....

Are there any recurring themes?

_____
_____
_____
_____
_____

How would you draw your dream?

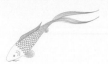

How would you interpret this dream?

Any related memories from the day before?

What was the moon phase?

Title: _____ Date/Time: _____ Location: _____

How did it make you feel?

☐ Excited   ☐ Overwhelmed   ☐ Anxious
☐ Happy   ☐ Confused   ☐ Scared
☐ Emotional   ☐ Worried   ☐ Vulnerable
☐ Relaxed   ☐ Frustrated   ☐ ....

Are there any recurring themes?

_____
_____
_____
_____
_____

How would you draw your dream?

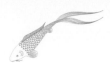

How would you interpret this dream?

Any related memories from the day before?

_____

_____

_____

_____

_____

What was the moon phase?

Title: _____ Date/Time: _____ Location: _____

How did it make you feel?

Are there any recurring themes?

☐ Excited ☐ Overwhelmed ☐ Anxious
☐ Happy ☐ Confused ☐ Scared
☐ Emotional ☐ Worried ☐ Vulnerable
☐ Relaxed ☐ Frustrated ☐ ....

_____
_____
_____
_____
_____

How would you draw your dream?

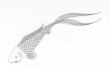

How would you interpret this dream?

Any related memories from the day before?

_____

_____

_____

_____

_____

What was the moon phase?

Title: _____ Date/Time: _____ Location: _____

How did it make you feel?

☐ Excited   ☐ Overwhelmed   ☐ Anxious
☐ Happy   ☐ Confused   ☐ Scared
☐ Emotional   ☐ Worried   ☐ Vulnerable
☐ Relaxed   ☐ Frustrated   ☐ ....

Are there any recurring themes?

_____
_____
_____
_____
_____

How would you draw your dream?

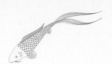

How would you interpret this dream?

Any related memories from the day before?

What was the moon phase?

Title: _____ Date/Time: _____ Location: _____

How did it make you feel?

☐	Excited	☐	Overwhelmed	☐	Anxious
☐	Happy	☐	Confused	☐	Scared
☐	Emotional	☐	Worried	☐	Vulnerable
☐	Relaxed	☐	Frustrated	☐	....

Are there any recurring themes?

_____
_____
_____
_____
_____

How would you draw your dream?

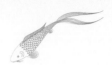

How would you interpret this dream?

Any related memories from the day before?

What was the moon phase?

Title: _____ Date/Time: _____ Location: _____

How did it make you feel?

☐ Excited   ☐ Overwhelmed   ☐ Anxious
☐ Happy   ☐ Confused   ☐ Scared
☐ Emotional   ☐ Worried   ☐ Vulnerable
☐ Relaxed   ☐ Frustrated   ☐ ....

Are there any recurring themes?

_____
_____
_____
_____
_____

Title: _____ Date/Time: _____ Location: _____

How did it make you feel?

☐ Excited   ☐ Overwhelmed   ☐ Anxious

☐ Happy   ☐ Confused   ☐ Scared

☐ Emotional   ☐ Worried   ☐ Vulnerable

☐ Relaxed   ☐ Frustrated   ☐ ....

Are there any recurring themes?

_____
_____
_____
_____
_____

Title: _____ Date/Time: _____ Location: _____

How did it make you feel?

☐ Excited   ☐ Overwhelmed   ☐ Anxious
☐ Happy   ☐ Confused   ☐ Scared
☐ Emotional   ☐ Worried   ☐ Vulnerable
☐ Relaxed   ☐ Frustrated   ☐ ....

Are there any recurring themes?

_____
_____
_____
_____
_____

Title: _____ Date/Time: _____ Location: _____

How did it make you feel?

☐ Excited   ☐ Overwhelmed   ☐ Anxious
☐ Happy   ☐ Confused   ☐ Scared
☐ Emotional   ☐ Worried   ☐ Vulnerable
☐ Relaxed   ☐ Frustrated   ☐ ....

Are there any recurring themes?

_____
_____
_____
_____
_____

Title: _____ Date/Time: _____ Location: _____

How did it make you feel?

☐ Excited
☐ Happy
☐ Emotional
☐ Relaxed

☐ Overwhelmed
☐ Confused
☐ Worried
☐ Frustrated

☐ Anxious
☐ Scared
☐ Vulnerable
☐ ....

Are there any recurring themes?

_____
_____
_____
_____
_____

Title: _____ Date/Time: _____ Location: _____

How did it make you feel?

Are there any recurring themes?

☐ Excited   ☐ Overwhelmed   ☐ Anxious
☐ Happy   ☐ Confused   ☐ Scared
☐ Emotional ☐ Worried   ☐ Vulnerable
☐ Relaxed   ☐ Frustrated   ☐ ....

_____
_____
_____
_____
_____

Title: _____ Date/Time: _____ Location: _____

How did it make you feel?

- [ ] Excited
- [ ] Happy
- [ ] Emotional
- [ ] Relaxed
- [ ] Overwhelmed
- [ ] Confused
- [ ] Worried
- [ ] Frustrated
- [ ] Anxious
- [ ] Scared
- [ ] Vulnerable
- [ ] ....

Are there any recurring themes?

_____
_____
_____
_____
_____

Title: _____ Date/Time: _____ Location: _____

How did it make you feel?

☐ Excited ☐ Overwhelmed ☐ Anxious
☐ Happy ☐ Confused ☐ Scared
☐ Emotional ☐ Worried ☐ Vulnerable
☐ Relaxed ☐ Frustrated ☐ ....

Are there any recurring themes?

_____
_____
_____
_____
_____

Title: _____ Date/Time: _____ Location: _____

How did it make you feel?

Are there any recurring themes?

- [ ] Excited
- [ ] Happy
- [ ] Emotional
- [ ] Relaxed

- [ ] Overwhelmed
- [ ] Confused
- [ ] Worried
- [ ] Frustrated

- [ ] Anxious
- [ ] Scared
- [ ] Vulnerable
- [ ] ....

_____
_____
_____
_____
_____

Title: _____ Date/Time: _____ Location: _____

How did it make you feel?

Are there any recurring themes?

- [ ] Excited
- [ ] Happy
- [ ] Emotional
- [ ] Relaxed
- [ ] Overwhelmed
- [ ] Confused
- [ ] Worried
- [ ] Frustrated
- [ ] Anxious
- [ ] Scared
- [ ] Vulnerable
- [ ] ....

_____
_____
_____
_____
_____

Title: _____ Date/Time: _____ Location: _____

How did it make you feel?

Are there any recurring themes?

☐ Excited   ☐ Overwhelmed   ☐ Anxious

☐ Happy   ☐ Confused   ☐ Scared

☐ Emotional   ☐ Worried   ☐ Vulnerable

☐ Relaxed   ☐ Frustrated   ☐ ....

_____
_____
_____
_____
_____

Title: _____ Date/Time: _____ Location: _____

How did it make you feel?

- [ ] Excited
- [ ] Happy
- [ ] Emotional
- [ ] Relaxed

- [ ] Overwhelmed
- [ ] Confused
- [ ] Worried
- [ ] Frustrated

- [ ] Anxious
- [ ] Scared
- [ ] Vulnerable
- [ ] ....

Are there any recurring themes?

_____
_____
_____
_____
_____

Title: _____ Date/Time: _____ Location: _____

How did it make you feel?

☐ Excited   ☐ Overwhelmed   ☐ Anxious
☐ Happy   ☐ Confused   ☐ Scared
☐ Emotional   ☐ Worried   ☐ Vulnerable
☐ Relaxed   ☐ Frustrated   ☐ ....

Are there any recurring themes?

_____
_____
_____
_____
_____

Title: _____ Date/Time: _____ Location: _____

How did it make you feel?

☐ Excited   ☐ Overwhelmed   ☐ Anxious
☐ Happy   ☐ Confused   ☐ Scared
☐ Emotional   ☐ Worried   ☐ Vulnerable
☐ Relaxed   ☐ Frustrated   ☐ ....

Are there any recurring themes?

_____
_____
_____
_____
_____

Title: _____   Date/Time: _____   Location: _____

How did it make you feel?   Are there any recurring themes?

☐ Excited   ☐ Overwhelmed   ☐ Anxious   _____
☐ Happy   ☐ Confused   ☐ Scared   _____
☐ Emotional   ☐ Worried   ☐ Vulnerable   _____
☐ Relaxed   ☐ Frustrated   ☐ ....   _____
                                                          _____

Title: _____ Date/Time: _____ Location: _____

How did it make you feel?

Are there any recurring themes?

☐ Excited   ☐ Overwhelmed   ☐ Anxious
☐ Happy   ☐ Confused   ☐ Scared
☐ Emotional ☐ Worried   ☐ Vulnerable
☐ Relaxed   ☐ Frustrated   ☐ ....

_____
_____
_____
_____
_____

Title: _____ Date/Time: _____ Location: _____

How did it make you feel?

☐ Excited ☐ Overwhelmed ☐ Anxious
☐ Happy ☐ Confused ☐ Scared
☐ Emotional ☐ Worried ☐ Vulnerable
☐ Relaxed ☐ Frustrated ☐ ....

Are there any recurring themes?

_____
_____
_____
_____
_____

Title: _____   Date/Time: _____   Location: _____

How did it make you feel?

☐ Excited	☐ Overwhelmed	☐ Anxious
☐ Happy	☐ Confused	☐ Scared
☐ Emotional	☐ Worried	☐ Vulnerable
☐ Relaxed	☐ Frustrated	☐ ....

Are there any recurring themes?

_____
_____
_____
_____
_____

Title: _____ Date/Time: _____ Location: _____

How did it make you feel?

- [ ] Excited
- [ ] Happy
- [ ] Emotional
- [ ] Relaxed
- [ ] Overwhelmed
- [ ] Confused
- [ ] Worried
- [ ] Frustrated
- [ ] Anxious
- [ ] Scared
- [ ] Vulnerable
- [ ] ....

Are there any recurring themes?

_____
_____
_____
_____
_____

Title: _____ Date/Time: _____ Location: _____

How did it make you feel?

☐ Excited ☐ Overwhelmed ☐ Anxious
☐ Happy ☐ Confused ☐ Scared
☐ Emotional ☐ Worried ☐ Vulnerable
☐ Relaxed ☐ Frustrated ☐ ....

Are there any recurring themes?

_____
_____
_____
_____
_____

Title: _____ Date/Time: _____ Location: _____

How did it make you feel?

☐ Excited   ☐ Overwhelmed   ☐ Anxious
☐ Happy   ☐ Confused   ☐ Scared
☐ Emotional   ☐ Worried   ☐ Vulnerable
☐ Relaxed   ☐ Frustrated   ☐ ....

Are there any recurring themes?

_____
_____
_____
_____
_____

Title: _____ Date/Time: _____ Location: _____

How did it make you feel?

☐ Excited
☐ Happy
☐ Emotional
☐ Relaxed

☐ Overwhelmed
☐ Confused
☐ Worried
☐ Frustrated

☐ Anxious
☐ Scared
☐ Vulnerable
☐ ....

Are there any recurring themes?

_____
_____
_____
_____
_____

Title: _____ Date/Time: _____ Location: _____

How did it make you feel?

☐ Excited   ☐ Overwhelmed   ☐ Anxious
☐ Happy   ☐ Confused   ☐ Scared
☐ Emotional ☐ Worried   ☐ Vulnerable
☐ Relaxed   ☐ Frustrated   ☐ ....

Are there any recurring themes?

_____
_____
_____
_____
_____

Title: _____ Date/Time: _____ Location: _____

How did it make you feel?

☐ Excited	☐ Overwhelmed	☐ Anxious
☐ Happy	☐ Confused	☐ Scared
☐ Emotional	☐ Worried	☐ Vulnerable
☐ Relaxed	☐ Frustrated	☐ ....

Are there any recurring themes?

_____
_____
_____
_____
_____

Title: _____ Date/Time: _____ Location: _____

How did it make you feel?

Are there any recurring themes?

☐ Excited	☐ Overwhelmed
☐ Happy	☐ Confused
☐ Emotional	☐ Worried
☐ Relaxed	☐ Frustrated

☐ Anxious
☐ Scared
☐ Vulnerable
☐ ....

_____
_____
_____
_____
_____

Title: _____ Date/Time: _____ Location: _____

How did it make you feel?

Are there any recurring themes?

☐ Excited	☐ Overwhelmed
☐ Happy	☐ Confused
☐ Emotional	☐ Worried
☐ Relaxed	☐ Frustrated

☐ Anxious
☐ Scared
☐ Vulnerable
☐ ....

_____
_____
_____
_____
_____

Title: _____ Date/Time: _____ Location: _____

How did it make you feel?

☐ Excited	☐ Overwhelmed	☐ Anxious
☐ Happy	☐ Confused	☐ Scared
☐ Emotional	☐ Worried	☐ Vulnerable
☐ Relaxed	☐ Frustrated	☐ ....

Are there any recurring themes?

_____
_____
_____
_____
_____

Title: _____ Date/Time: _____ Location: _____

How did it make you feel?

☐ Excited	☐ Overwhelmed	☐ Anxious
☐ Happy	☐ Confused	☐ Scared
☐ Emotional	☐ Worried	☐ Vulnerable
☐ Relaxed	☐ Frustrated	☐ ....

Are there any recurring themes?

_____
_____
_____
_____
_____

Title: _____ Date/Time: _____ Location: _____

How did it make you feel?

Are there any recurring themes?

☐ Excited ☐ Overwhelmed ☐ Anxious

☐ Happy ☐ Confused ☐ Scared

☐ Emotional ☐ Worried ☐ Vulnerable

☐ Relaxed ☐ Frustrated ☐ ....

_____

_____

_____

_____

_____

Title: _____ Date/Time: _____ Location: _____

How did it make you feel?

☐ Excited   ☐ Overwhelmed   ☐ Anxious
☐ Happy   ☐ Confused   ☐ Scared
☐ Emotional   ☐ Worried   ☐ Vulnerable
☐ Relaxed   ☐ Frustrated   ☐ ....

Are there any recurring themes?

_____
_____
_____
_____
_____

Title: _____ Date/Time: _____ Location: _____

How did it make you feel?

Are there any recurring themes?

☐ Excited   ☐ Overwhelmed   ☐ Anxious

☐ Happy   ☐ Confused   ☐ Scared

☐ Emotional   ☐ Worried   ☐ Vulnerable

☐ Relaxed   ☐ Frustrated   ☐ ....

_____

_____

_____

_____

_____

Title: _____ Date/Time: _____ Location: _____

How did it make you feel?

☐ Excited   ☐ Overwhelmed   ☐ Anxious
☐ Happy   ☐ Confused   ☐ Scared
☐ Emotional   ☐ Worried   ☐ Vulnerable
☐ Relaxed   ☐ Frustrated   ☐ ....

Are there any recurring themes?

_____
_____
_____
_____
_____

Title: _____ Date/Time: _____ Location: _____

How did it make you feel?

Are there any recurring themes?

☐ Excited   ☐ Overwhelmed   ☐ Anxious
☐ Happy   ☐ Confused   ☐ Scared
☐ Emotional ☐ Worried   ☐ Vulnerable
☐ Relaxed   ☐ Frustrated   ☐ ....

_____
_____
_____
_____
_____

Title: _____ Date/Time: _____ Location: _____

How did it make you feel?

- [ ] Excited
- [ ] Happy
- [ ] Emotional
- [ ] Relaxed

- [ ] Overwhelmed
- [ ] Confused
- [ ] Worried
- [ ] Frustrated

- [ ] Anxious
- [ ] Scared
- [ ] Vulnerable
- [ ] ....

Are there any recurring themes?

_____
_____
_____
_____
_____

Title: _____ Date/Time: _____ Location: _____

How did it make you feel?

- [ ] Excited
- [ ] Happy
- [ ] Emotional
- [ ] Relaxed

- [ ] Overwhelmed
- [ ] Confused
- [ ] Worried
- [ ] Frustrated

- [ ] Anxious
- [ ] Scared
- [ ] Vulnerable
- [ ] ....

Are there any recurring themes?

_____
_____
_____
_____
_____

Title: _____ Date/Time: _____ Location: _____

How did it make you feel?

Are there any recurring themes?

	Excited		Overwhelmed		Anxious
	Happy		Confused		Scared
	Emotional		Worried		Vulnerable
	Relaxed		Frustrated		....

_____
_____
_____
_____
_____

Title: _____ Date/Time: _____ Location: _____

How did it make you feel?

☐ Excited   ☐ Overwhelmed   ☐ Anxious
☐ Happy   ☐ Confused   ☐ Scared
☐ Emotional   ☐ Worried   ☐ Vulnerable
☐ Relaxed   ☐ Frustrated   ☐ ....

Are there any recurring themes?

_____
_____
_____
_____
_____

Title: _____ Date/Time: _____ Location: _____

How did it make you feel?

☐ Excited	☐ Overwhelmed
☐ Happy	☐ Confused
☐ Emotional	☐ Worried
☐ Relaxed	☐ Frustrated

☐ Anxious
☐ Scared
☐ Vulnerable
☐ ....

Are there any recurring themes?

_____
_____
_____
_____
_____

Title: _____ Date/Time: _____ Location: _____

How did it make you feel?

☐ Excited ☐ Overwhelmed ☐ Anxious
☐ Happy ☐ Confused ☐ Scared
☐ Emotional ☐ Worried ☐ Vulnerable
☐ Relaxed ☐ Frustrated ☐ ....

Are there any recurring themes?

_____
_____
_____
_____
_____

Title: _____ Date/Time: _____ Location: _____

How did it make you feel?

- [ ] Excited
- [ ] Happy
- [ ] Emotional
- [ ] Relaxed

- [ ] Overwhelmed
- [ ] Confused
- [ ] Worried
- [ ] Frustrated

- [ ] Anxious
- [ ] Scared
- [ ] Vulnerable
- [ ] ....

Are there any recurring themes?

_____
_____
_____
_____
_____

Title: _____ Date/Time: _____ Location: _____

How did it make you feel?

- [ ] Excited
- [ ] Happy
- [ ] Emotional
- [ ] Relaxed
- [ ] Overwhelmed
- [ ] Confused
- [ ] Worried
- [ ] Frustrated
- [ ] Anxious
- [ ] Scared
- [ ] Vulnerable
- [ ] ....

Are there any recurring themes?

_____
_____
_____
_____
_____

Title: _____ Date/Time: _____ Location: _____

How did it make you feel?

☐ Excited   ☐ Overwhelmed   ☐ Anxious
☐ Happy   ☐ Confused   ☐ Scared
☐ Emotional   ☐ Worried   ☐ Vulnerable
☐ Relaxed   ☐ Frustrated   ☐ ....

Are there any recurring themes?

_____
_____
_____
_____
_____

Title: _____ Date/Time: _____ Location: _____

How did it make you feel?

☐ Excited   ☐ Overwhelmed   ☐ Anxious

☐ Happy   ☐ Confused   ☐ Scared

☐ Emotional   ☐ Worried   ☐ Vulnerable

☐ Relaxed   ☐ Frustrated   ☐ ....

Are there any recurring themes?

_____

_____

_____

_____

_____

Title: _____ Date/Time: _____ Location: _____

How did it make you feel?

- [ ] Excited
- [ ] Happy
- [ ] Emotional
- [ ] Relaxed

- [ ] Overwhelmed
- [ ] Confused
- [ ] Worried
- [ ] Frustrated

- [ ] Anxious
- [ ] Scared
- [ ] Vulnerable
- [ ] ....

Are there any recurring themes?

_____
_____
_____
_____
_____

Title: _____ Date/Time: _____ Location: _____

How did it make you feel?

Are there any recurring themes?

- [ ] Excited
- [ ] Happy
- [ ] Emotional
- [ ] Relaxed

- [ ] Overwhelmed
- [ ] Confused
- [ ] Worried
- [ ] Frustrated

- [ ] Anxious
- [ ] Scared
- [ ] Vulnerable
- [ ] ....

_____
_____
_____
_____
_____

Title: _____ Date/Time: _____ Location: _____

How did it make you feel?

☐ Excited ☐ Overwhelmed ☐ Anxious
☐ Happy ☐ Confused ☐ Scared
☐ Emotional ☐ Worried ☐ Vulnerable
☐ Relaxed ☐ Frustrated ☐ ....

Are there any recurring themes?

_____
_____
_____
_____
_____

Title: _____   Date/Time: _____   Location: _____

How did it make you feel?

☐ Excited	☐ Overwhelmed	☐ Anxious
☐ Happy	☐ Confused	☐ Scared
☐ Emotional	☐ Worried	☐ Vulnerable
☐ Relaxed	☐ Frustrated	☐ ....

Are there any recurring themes?

_____

_____

_____

_____

_____

Title: _____ Date/Time: _____ Location: _____

How did it make you feel?

☐ Excited   ☐ Overwhelmed   ☐ Anxious
☐ Happy   ☐ Confused   ☐ Scared
☐ Emotional ☐ Worried   ☐ Vulnerable
☐ Relaxed   ☐ Frustrated   ☐ ....

Are there any recurring themes?

_____
_____
_____
_____
_____

Title: _____ Date/Time: _____ Location: _____

How did it make you feel?

- [ ] Excited
- [ ] Happy
- [ ] Emotional
- [ ] Relaxed

- [ ] Overwhelmed
- [ ] Confused
- [ ] Worried
- [ ] Frustrated

- [ ] Anxious
- [ ] Scared
- [ ] Vulnerable
- [ ] ....

Are there any recurring themes?

_____
_____
_____
_____
_____

Title: _____ Date/Time: _____ Location: _____

How did it make you feel?

☐ Excited
☐ Happy
☐ Emotional
☐ Relaxed

☐ Overwhelmed
☐ Confused
☐ Worried
☐ Frustrated

☐ Anxious
☐ Scared
☐ Vulnerable
☐ ....

Are there any recurring themes?

_____
_____
_____
_____
_____

Title: _____ Date/Time: _____ Location: _____

How did it make you feel?

☐ Excited	☐ Overwhelmed	☐ Anxious			
☐ Happy	☐ Confused	☐ Scared			
☐ Emotional	☐ Worried	☐ Vulnerable			
☐ Relaxed	☐ Frustrated	☐			

Are there any recurring themes?

_____
_____
_____
_____
_____

Title: _____ Date/Time: _____ Location: _____

How did it make you feel?

☐ Excited   ☐ Overwhelmed   ☐ Anxious
☐ Happy   ☐ Confused   ☐ Scared
☐ Emotional   ☐ Worried   ☐ Vulnerable
☐ Relaxed   ☐ Frustrated   ☐ ....

Are there any recurring themes?

_____
_____
_____
_____
_____

Title: _____ Date/Time: _____ Location: _____

How did it make you feel?

☐ Excited ☐ Overwhelmed ☐ Anxious
☐ Happy ☐ Confused ☐ Scared
☐ Emotional ☐ Worried ☐ Vulnerable
☐ Relaxed ☐ Frustrated ☐ ....

Are there any recurring themes?

_____
_____
_____
_____
_____

Title: _____ Date/Time: _____ Location: _____

How did it make you feel?

	Excited		Overwhelmed		Anxious
	Happy		Confused		Scared
	Emotional		Worried		Vulnerable
	Relaxed		Frustrated		....

Are there any recurring themes?

_____
_____
_____
_____
_____

Title: _____ Date/Time: _____ Location: _____

How did it make you feel?

☐ Excited	☐ Overwhelmed	☐ Anxious
☐ Happy	☐ Confused	☐ Scared
☐ Emotional	☐ Worried	☐ Vulnerable
☐ Relaxed	☐ Frustrated	☐ ....

Are there any recurring themes?

_____
_____
_____
_____
_____

Title: _____ Date/Time: _____ Location: _____

How did it make you feel?

- [ ] Excited
- [ ] Happy
- [ ] Emotional
- [ ] Relaxed

- [ ] Overwhelmed
- [ ] Confused
- [ ] Worried
- [ ] Frustrated

- [ ] Anxious
- [ ] Scared
- [ ] Vulnerable
- [ ] ....

Are there any recurring themes?

_____
_____
_____
_____
_____

Title: _____ Date/Time: _____ Location: _____

How did it make you feel?

☐ Excited	☐ Overwhelmed	☐ Anxious
☐ Happy	☐ Confused	☐ Scared
☐ Emotional	☐ Worried	☐ Vulnerable
☐ Relaxed	☐ Frustrated	☐ ....

Are there any recurring themes?

_____
_____
_____
_____
_____

Title: _____ Date/Time: _____ Location: _____

How did it make you feel?

☐ Excited   ☐ Overwhelmed   ☐ Anxious
☐ Happy   ☐ Confused   ☐ Scared
☐ Emotional   ☐ Worried   ☐ Vulnerable
☐ Relaxed   ☐ Frustrated   ☐ ....

Are there any recurring themes?

_____
_____
_____
_____
_____

Title: _____ Date/Time: _____ Location: _____

How did it make you feel?

- [ ] Excited
- [ ] Happy
- [ ] Emotional
- [ ] Relaxed

- [ ] Overwhelmed
- [ ] Confused
- [ ] Worried
- [ ] Frustrated

- [ ] Anxious
- [ ] Scared
- [ ] Vulnerable
- [ ] ....

Are there any recurring themes?

_____
_____
_____
_____
_____

Title: _____ Date/Time: _____ Location: _____

How did it make you feel?

☐ Excited	☐ Overwhelmed	☐ Anxious
☐ Happy	☐ Confused	☐ Scared
☐ Emotional	☐ Worried	☐ Vulnerable
☐ Relaxed	☐ Frustrated	☐ ....

Are there any recurring themes?

_____
_____
_____
_____
_____

Title: _____ Date/Time: _____ Location: _____

How did it make you feel?

	Excited		Overwhelmed		Anxious
	Happy		Confused		Scared
	Emotional		Worried		Vulnerable
	Relaxed		Frustrated		....

Are there any recurring themes?

_____
_____
_____
_____
_____

Title: _____ Date/Time: _____ Location: _____

How did it make you feel?

Are there any recurring themes?

☐ Excited   ☐ Overwhelmed   ☐ Anxious
☐ Happy   ☐ Confused   ☐ Scared
☐ Emotional   ☐ Worried   ☐ Vulnerable
☐ Relaxed   ☐ Frustrated   ☐ ....

_____
_____
_____
_____
_____

Title: _____ Date/Time: _____ Location: _____

Title: _____ Date/Time: _____ Location: _____

Title: _____ Date/Time: _____ Location: _____

Title: _____ Date/Time: _____ Location: _____

Title: _____ Date/Time: _____ Location: _____

Title: _____ Date/Time: _____ Location: _____

Title: _____ Date/Time: _____ Location: _____

Title: _____ Date/Time: _____ Location: _____

Title: _____ Date/Time: _____ Location: _____

Title: _____ Date/Time: _____ Location: _____

Title: _____ Date/Time: _____ Location: _____

Title: _____ Date/Time: _____ Location: _____

Title: _____ Date/Time: _____ Location: _____

Title: _____ Date/Time: _____ Location: _____

Title: _____ Date/Time: _____ Location: _____

Title: _____ Date/Time: _____ Location: _____

Title: _____ Date/Time: _____ Location: _____

Title: _____ Date/Time: _____ Location: _____

Title: _____ Date/Time: _____ Location: _____

Title: _____ Date/Time: _____ Location: _____

Title: _____ Date/Time: _____ Location: _____

Title: _____ Date/Time: _____ Location: _____

Title: _____ Date/Time: _____ Location: _____

Title: _____ Date/Time: _____ Location: _____

HOW TO INTERPRET YOUR DREAMS

When you feel ready to revisit your dream, grab your dream journal and find somewhere quiet where you won't be disturbed. Take a few deep breaths, then slowly and carefully reread your dream entries. As you read, be aware that your dreams don't speak to you in the language of your waking life—they speak to you in the language of symbols, and those symbols will be personal to you. For example, if you love dogs and dream of a dog, this may suggest loyalty and unconditional love; if you are afraid of dogs, your dream dog may suggest something about yourself and your life that is menacing. As you ponder the symbols you have recorded in your journal, look for the following:

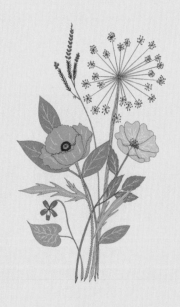

Your role

Who, what, when, and where were you in the dream? Did you appear in your dream or were you observing? If you did appear, did you recognize yourself or were you acting out of character?

Other people and things

Be aware that everyone and everything in your dream represents an aspect of yourself and your life. So, if you dreamed of a family member, loved one, friend, or colleague, you are not actually dreaming about them but rather those aspects of your character they represent, which you need to acknowledge, express, or come to terms with.

Feelings

If you are struggling to uncover the meaning of a dream, focus your interpretation on the feelings your dream inspires in you. Feelings are often the greatest teacher.

Motion

If your dream features movement of any kind this is symbolic of your progress through life. Are you flying or falling? Are you moving with ease or wading through mud? Are you rushing closer to something, someone, or somewhere, or are you floating or running away? If you are moving in a vehicle, are you in the driver's seat or is someone else driving you? Do you even know where you are going?

Waking life

What symbols, feelings, and images comment on or relate to your waking life?

Recurring themes

If you notice recurring symbols, images, and feelings in your dreams, especially if those patterns repeat over several weeks or months, take careful note: your dreaming mind is really trying to get your attention. You may find that these elements will keep recurring until you are able to understand them.

When you have had a chance to reflect on these areas, have a go at writing down your own interpretation. Does it sound plausible? Does it prompt any further insight?

A DICTIONARY
OF DREAMS

ANXIETY

BEING LATE..130

BEING LOST/LOSING SOMETHING...130

BEING UNPREPARED...131

CAR OUT OF CONTROL OR SPEEDING...131

CHEATING ON A PARTNER...132

FALLING..132

FEELING TRAPPED...133

NUDITY..133

PARALYSIS..134

ROBOTS/ALIENS...134

TEETH FALLING OUT..135

UNABLE TO FIND A BATHROOM...135

CRISIS

ACCIDENTS...136

APOCALYPSE...136

BEING CHASED..137

DEATH OR DYING...137

DEMON OR MONSTER..138

DISASTERS...138

DROWNING..139

FIRE...139

INTRUDERS...140

MURDER...140

NATURE

ANIMALS..141

BIRDS...141

FLOWERS...142

INSECTS/REPTILES..142

TREES/MOUNTAINS/GARDENS...143

WATER...143

OBJECTS

BODY PARTS..144

BOOKS/WRITING/WORDS...144

CELL PHONES...145

CLOTHES...145

FOOD OR DRINK...146
MONEY...146
MUSICAL INSTRUMENTS...147
NUMBERS...147
SHOPPING..148
SOCIAL MEDIA...148
TECHNOLOGY...149
TRANSPORT..149

PEOPLE/RELATIONSHIPS
ACTOR/CELEBRITY..150
BABY/BIRTH..150
CHILDREN..151
DECEASED PEOPLE..151
ELDERLY PEOPLE...152
FAMILY..152
PEOPLE...153
RELIGIOUS OR SPIRITUAL FIGURES...153
SEX..154
WEDDING/MARRIAGE..154

PLACES
BEACH...155
BUILDINGS...155
CASTLES/ANCIENT BUILDINGS/TOMBS...156
SCHOOL..156
UNFAMILIAR, SECRET, OR UNUSED ROOM...157
WORK..157

POSITIVE EXPERIENCES
FINDING SOMETHING VALUABLE..158
FLYING WITHOUT WINGS..158
MOVING FORWARD..159
SUPERHERO POWERS...159

BEING LATE

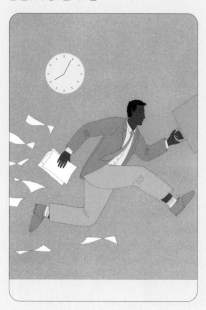

Turning up late for an appointment or event can have a range of possible meanings, usually on the theme of something problematic in your approach to some aspect of your life. Perhaps you're showing a lack of confidence or self-esteem or not dealing effectively with practical matters. The most common manifestation is missing a flight or a train—a classic symbol of feeling overwhelmed or not up to the challenge of a task. An alternative meaning is loss of control—in particular, perhaps, an inability to cope with deadlines or time pressures. Turning up late in general may be an alert suggesting you need to be more organized and disciplined. But sometimes it's a nudge to make you face your fears and deal with a situation you've been avoiding. If you've suffered a loss of some kind, being late may be, straightforwardly, a reflection of sorrow or regret.

BEING LOST/LOSING SOMETHING

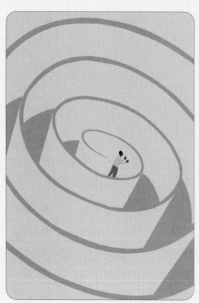

Dreams about being lost, or trying and failing to find something or someone, are obviously anxiety related. In waking life you may be feeling confused or directionless, or that you don't fit in or aren't up to a task or situation. The dream should prompt you to take an honest look at your life to identify what's causing such feelings. If you lose someone you know in a dream, perhaps he or she represents aspects of yourself you feel you're losing touch with. Losing keys or a phone may symbolize a sense of exclusion. If the lost item is precious or indispensable, it could stand in for a broken or interrupted relationship. Perhaps you need to give yourself time to grieve, let go, and heal before you can move forward. Dreams of abandonment tend to have similar meanings, since loss is often perceived as abandonment at a deep psychological level.

BEING UNPREPARED

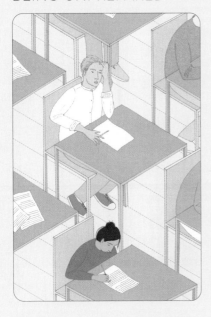

Being unprepared for an exam or important event, or taking and failing a test, suggests you aren't meeting the standards you've set for yourself. It may appear in the dream that you're being judged by teachers, instructors, or interviewers, but in reality it's you who are judging yourself—harshly. You may lack self-esteem as well as being worried that you are falling short of others' expectations. Your dreaming mind wants you to feel more confident and live life on your own terms. It's prompting you to focus more on your strengths than your weaknesses. If, of course, the dream corresponds literally with a real-life situation, it's simply reflecting your anxiety about being ill-prepared. Sometimes a dream will take an episode from your past, such as school days or college, and use it to address your current situation—don't imagine it's simply a case of old worries resurfacing.

CAR OUT OF CONTROL OR SPEEDING

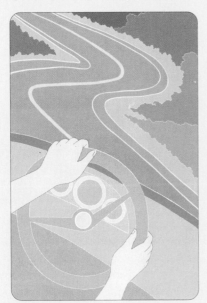

Cars represent your path in life or the direction you're currently taking. An out-of-control or speeding car suggests you might be veering off track or moving faster than you should. You may be heading for danger in some area of life—for example, rushing with not enough thought into a new relationship (or leaving an established one) or plunging too hastily into a big life change, such as a new job or a relocation (although the warning could be about something less serious, like a vacation plan). If you aren't the driver, the dream may be telling you that you ought to be: someone may be leading you astray, or perhaps you're being influenced by another's agenda. A driverless car often points to powerlessness, a sense of aimless drifting. If this interpretation seems probable, try to identify the forces that control you and consider how to regain the initiative.

CHEATING ON A PARTNER

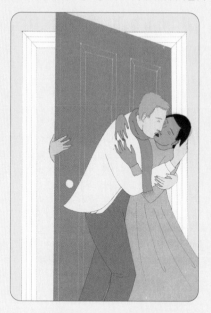

Dreams of sexual cheating in which you are the betrayer are rarely about you cheating in real life. They are often an indication that your relationship needs aren't being met in some way. You might be feeling neglected or fearful your partner may abandon or betray you. If you're the guilty party in the dream, pay attention to who you're having an affair with. Contrary to popular belief, this is not a wish-fulfillment dream: sleeping with someone else probably means there's some aspect of their personality you need to assimilate within yourself. If you don't know the person, this indicates that you feel something is missing from your current relationship or your life in general—excitement perhaps. If you dream your partner is cheating, the likely interpretation is more obvious, relating to your own feelings of insecurity, or of being sidelined in some way that you need to address in real life.

FALLING

TOP 10 DREAM

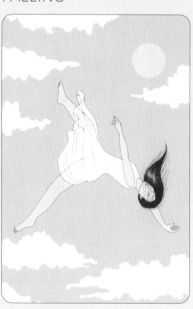

Falling in a dream is a clear sign that some situation or relationship is out of your control. It's unlikely to be significant whether you fall from a cliff, roof, plane, building, or other high place. Whatever the precise scenario, you find yourself with nothing to hold on to: you have no sense of stability. The key theme of this dream is insecurity. It may be that you see no solution to your problems (for example, low self-esteem), have too little support, or have a strong urge to escape a challenging situation. If the latter, the dream may be warning you to take control before you become too reckless and make a serious mistake—as in the popular expression, "You're heading for a fall." There may also be sexual associations—perhaps a strong desire to succumb to sexual urges, with a risk of damaging consequences.

FEELING TRAPPED

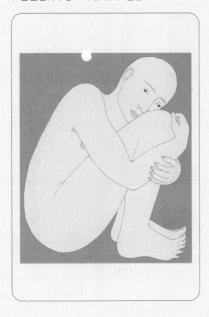

Feeling trapped, crushed, imprisoned, confined, or buried alive in a dream are variants of a theme that normally carries the same meaning: **you feel someone or something is squeezing the vitality out of you or holding you back in waking life.** Not even being able to scream suggests that your voice is not being heard. The dream may indicate that you've intuitively understood your situation, have looked at possible options, and have been unable to find a way out—in other words, part of being stuck is to do with indecision. Confinement dreams can also be a way for your unconscious to tell you that some of your patterns of thought or action are somehow impeding personal progress. This might, of course, be to do with a relationship. This kind of dream is often a potent wake-up call. You need to reevaluate and refresh: it's time to find new ways to move forward.

NUDITY

TOP 10 DREAM

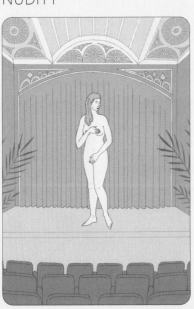

Being naked or nude, or partially clothed, is a strong indicator of feeling vulnerable in your waking life. Perhaps you're hiding something or not being true to who you really are. You might feel anxious that others will see through your disguise. Or you might be trying hard to impress but afraid you'll cause disappointment. The dream may be highlighting a tension: on the one hand, you want to be completely honest and open with people (or someone in particular); on the other, you're afraid that if you do reveal your true feelings or personality, you'll be ridiculed or exposed as a fraud. The reaction of others to your nudity (as well as your own reaction) will help to clarify the dream's meaning. If you don't feel embarrassed, perhaps you're being encouraged to be proud of who you are, or the way you think or act. If other people don't notice your nakedness, maybe you're worrying needlessly.

PARALYSIS

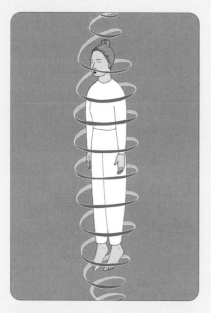

Dreams in which you can't move or speak can cause great anxiety. The simplest explanation is that you feel helpless and trapped in some aspect of your life. For some reason you're unable to move forward, perhaps because you can't decide on the best course of action. If you're disabled in a dream, or a wheelchair or disabled person appears, this may reflect an aspect of yourself that's struggling to express itself or realize its potential. Perhaps you're lacking confidence or have ambitions or goals you feel are beyond you. A situation may not have worked out as you'd hoped. Alternatively, someone may have hurt you badly, in a way you might not even have acknowledged to yourself. If your immobility results from being weighed down with heavy bags, this is a sign of taking on too many responsibilities: you might need to say "no" more often or ask others to help you.

ROBOTS/ALIENS

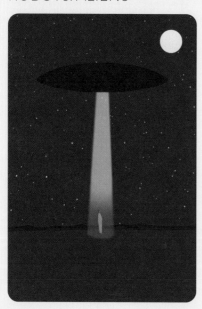

Aliens and/or UFOs in a dream may indicate your desire to escape reality. Perhaps your mind is visionary in character: your imagination can take you beyond the limits of the ordinary. The downside of this abundant creativity is that you may have problems fitting in with worldly expectations. There may be some lack of connection between yourself and others: you may feel different in some way and struggle to conform to the requirements of a role. This kind of dream is urging you to celebrate your uniqueness. It may also suggest that there are aspects of yourself you have yet to discover. Dreams about robots may have a similar meaning, but expressed as a warning: you may be losing your individuality in your attempts to conform. Alternatively, you may need to be more logical and less emotional in your daily life. Or could the opposite be true? The dream's mood may make this clearer.

TEETH FALLING OUT

TOP 10 DREAM

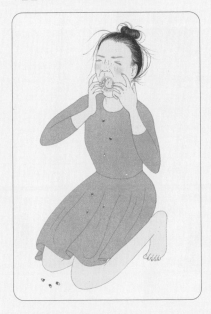

Teeth falling out may suggest fear of aging or feeling unattractive or unappealing in some way. It can also symbolize fear of losing something or someone important to your emotional or material survival—after all, without teeth you can't eat and nourish yourself. The tooth fairy association links this dream with money, too, so there may be a reference to financial concerns. Teeth are symbols of viability or, sometimes, power. Hence, this dream might suggest you're feeling neglected, frustrated, overlooked, or inferior in some way. Maybe there are basic actions you ought or want to take but can't because you're ill-equipped. It could be that this disturbing dream scenario wants to shock you into having more belief in yourself and being more assertive. It's also worth noting that in Chinese tradition teeth crumbling or falling out is associated with telling lies or not being true to yourself.

UNABLE TO FIND A BATHROOM

TOP 10 DREAM

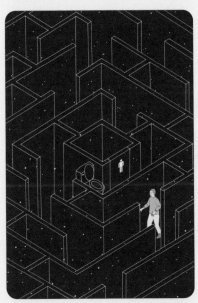

Searching unsuccessfully for a bathroom or lavatory is a sign you're feeling frustrated or blocked in some way in waking life. Since using a bathroom is a very personal thing to do, the dream is probably concerned with some deep aspect of your inner life. One possible message is that you need to let go of any anger, guilt, shame, jealousy, fear, hate, or sadness—emotion appears to be holding you back. Another is that you aren't paying enough attention to your life's true priorities or you're neglecting your personal needs. You're probably placing others' priorities above your own well-being and would be well advised to take better care of yourself. Give yourself more space, calm, respect, and freedom. If you do find the bathroom, this is a positive sign that you'll find a healthy way to let go—unless the room turns out to be unusable, in which case the warning still applies.

ACCIDENTS

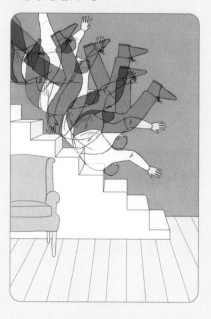

Dreams that feature accidents—perhaps in a car, plane, or train, or simply tripping up and falling over—are an obvious warning to be alert to potential danger. Your unconscious has noticed, and wants to draw your attention to, something you aren't alert to in waking life. It's urging you to be more careful. This doesn't mean you're going to have an accident, just that greater vigilance is required if you're to reach your goals without some kind of mischance, which may occur at the emotional level. Alternatively, the accident could suggest you're avoiding something you need to face or that your priorities or values are in conflict with those of others. If you're driving and crash, you may be experiencing strong emotions that put you in danger of losing control. If someone else is driving, you probably feel a situation in waking life has left you powerless to shape your destiny.

APOCALYPSE

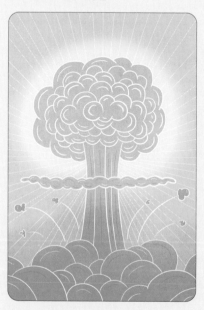

Contrary to what you might expect, a dream of the world ending is typically an exciting and positive sign, because brave new beginnings always follow. Apocalypse scenarios suggest that dramatic physical and/or emotional changes are taking place in your life or that they are urgently needed for you to reach your full potential. Courage will be called upon to live through these changes, but it will be well worth the effort as the outcome could be thrilling. You'll feel more fulfilled and more alive as a result, but to get to that awakened state your world as you currently experience it must be dismantled in some way. Even if the dream appears fearful in mood it will not usually be pointing to something you must avoid—only to the importance of letting go of the familiar and being strong enough to strike out in new directions.

BEING CHASED

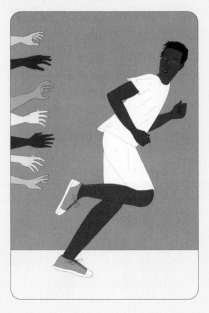

Being chased in a dream is a powerful indication you're trying to avoid someone or something in waking life. Running away or feeling the need to hide or escape usually carries the same meaning, even when no specific threat appears. When the identity of the threat is apparent, it may offer you clues, but if it remains vague, generalized, or unknown, as it often does, chances are it has an emotional source. Perhaps you're trying to deny or hide from painful feelings; or you may be running away from a responsibility or expectation, either self-imposed or placed upon you by others. If you continue to avoid dealing with the issue, there's a likelihood that this unsettling but common dream will recur. Such dreams can be hard to interpret, since they require a considerable degree of self-understanding; using a close friend as a sounding board can often help.

DEATH OR DYING

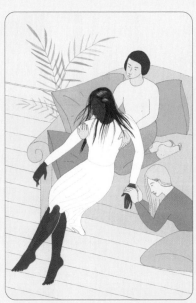

Death or dying are among the most commonly misinterpreted of all dream subjects. Contrary to popular belief, such dreams are not an omen that you or someone close to you is going to die—quite the opposite. Dreams about death are typically a sign of positive change, of shedding the past and moving forward. If you are dying in a dream, this suggests inner growth and self-discovery, or that you're starting a new phase in your life—for example, finishing a course of training or therapy. If someone else dies, this could mean simply that your relationship with this individual is evolving. Alternatively, the person who dies may represent an aspect of yourself that needs to be transformed: one phase needs to end and a new one be started. If you don't know the deceased, perhaps you're feeling removed from what's happening in your life, deep down, and need to do some serious self-examination.

DEMON OR MONSTER

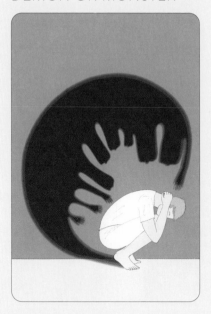

We all have our demons. When they appear in dreams, in some grotesque or scary form, they may represent emotions we've been repressing or hiding. An alien or monster in a dream can have a similar meaning. Your dreaming mind is encouraging you to come to terms with something that's inwardly plaguing or intimidating you. The problem may be an emotion such as anger, fear, or anxiety that has gotten out of control and morphed into a malevolent force. Alternatively, it might be a situation that's gotten out of hand, or a person who refuses to listen to you, respect you, or take your feelings or wishes into account. Maybe they have taken advantage of you, possibly by exploiting your good nature? Since monsters are a fiction, the dream could also be suggesting to your unconscious mind that you see your delusions for what they are and get "real."

DISASTERS

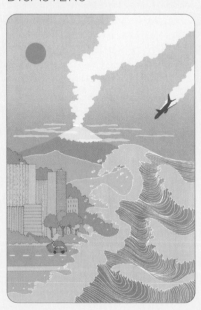

Dreaming of any kind of disaster, whether natural (earthquake, flood, fire) or man-made (explosion, bomb, accident), can be extremely unsettling. However, such dreams are not typically precognitive. They are more likely to suggest fears or anxieties, or something that you feel is out of your control. Perhaps you're anxious about your future or your peace of mind? Or possibly you're worried about your health? Alternatively, you may be going through a personal change that is making you feel uncertain about your direction in life. If the disaster has many victims, maybe your unconscious is telling you it's time to stop following the crowd. An avalanche may suggest you feel burdened down with responsibility or emotional pressure. Fire may suggest passion: perhaps your emotions are rampaging dangerously. An act of terrorism can reflect social insecurity, the feeling that others are not to be trusted or can't be understood.

DROWNING

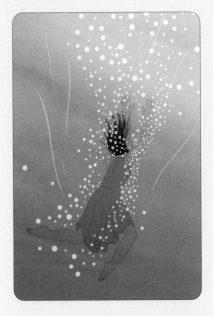

Water in dreams universally symbolizes emotions, so if you're drowning this indicates that you're either under a lot of emotional stress or afraid of being overcome by intense emotion. This dream may be a warning that something or someone is taking up too much of your energy and time. You might be too deeply immersed in a relationship or project and in danger of losing yourself. Perhaps you've overcommitted yourself at the expense of your health and well-being. Or you might simply have too many things going on in your life—for example, you might be juggling roles (parent, professional, volunteer, and so on) and consequently finding that you have too little quality time to yourself. If you're breathing underwater, this could indicate that you're navigating your way successfully through challenges. However, it could also symbolize a retreat to the womb, prompted by feelings of helplessness and dependency.

FIRE

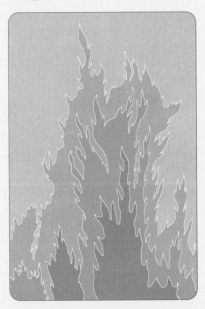

Fire—or fire-related images such as volcanoes, fireworks, burning, or smoking—probably indicates that you're experiencing passionate emotions in your waking life. Fire is purifying, illuminating, and the source of life, so it could suggest personal transformation or enlightenment. However, if you feel threatened or are injured in your dream, perhaps you're putting yourself at risk ("playing with fire"). Something urgently needs your attention before it gets out of control: it can't be ignored or avoided any longer, as it has the potential to be destructive. If you burn alive in a dream, maybe you're being overambitious or too driven, or too eager to impress. Maybe you need to take some time out to avoid burnout, especially in a professional context. If a firefighter or fire extinguisher appears, perhaps you're learning to control your emotions, even if you aren't yet doing so—so there's reason to have good hope of personal progress.

INTRUDERS

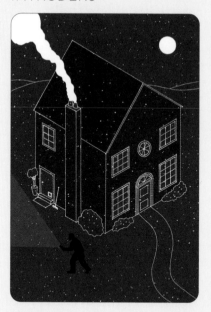

A house or home can represent your ego or inner world, so intruders or burglars usually indicate that a deep transformation is taking place or is needed. You may feel deeply insecure, especially if you don't know who the intruder is. Perhaps you need to take measures to build your confidence. There may be particular aspects of yourself you don't feel comfortable with; if so, acknowledge what they are and work out a way of dealing with them. A variation of this dream, carrying a similar meaning, is trying to hold a door shut to keep someone out, or knowing that someone else is in your house without your say-so. If you wake feeling anxious, this suggests the problem is quite severe—spend some time in self-reflection to identify what is troubling you deep down, and then ask yourself what steps are needed to find calm.

MURDER

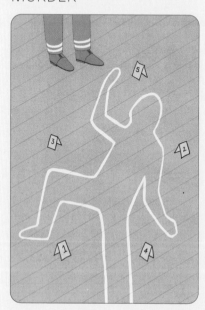

If you dream of a murder, violent death, or attack—perhaps a shooting, knifing, execution, or mugging—this may symbolize an aspect of yourself that isn't being expressed. If you're the perpetrator, pay attention to who the victim is, as this will represent an uncomfortable aspect of yourself you're denying and need to deal with—a clue about an internal conflict. If someone is trying to kill you, perhaps you're being affected in waking life by forces or elements over which you feel you have no control. Try to identify the attacker, as that will help you understand who or what is frustrating your progress. If you feel any kind of pain in your dream, this can indicate a fear of being hurt; alternatively, it may be a warning against taking unnecessary risks. If you're impaled or pierced, this suggests an unwanted intrusion into some aspect of your life.

ANIMALS

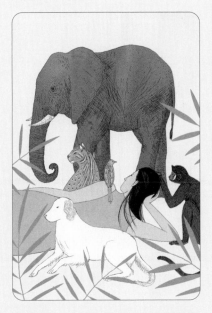

Animals are a symbol of primal instincts and urges. In a dream they can represent a repressed part of yourself that you can't fully express in waking life. The precise meaning may depend on the specific animal, so be alert to its character and its traditional associations. The most common wild animals to appear in dreams are the elephant, which denotes memories, or maybe a need for patience; the horse, which symbolizes strength or the need for that quality; and the lion, which suggests leadership and pride. If the animal is caged or in a zoo, you are being advised either to show caution or else to escape the constraints placed upon you—the mood of your dream may help you choose between these opposites. Pets, if they are healthy and content, suggest that your needs are being met, but a sick, wounded, or neglected pet suggests precisely the opposite.

BIRDS

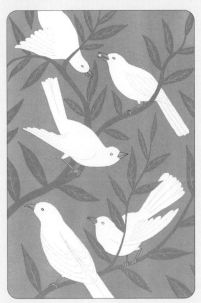

A bird or flock of birds is generally a positive sign—a symbol of freedom and joy as well as your hopes and aspirations taking flight. Pay attention to altitude: flying high can be taken metaphorically. The type of bird and its particular associations can be significant. Eagles, hawks, falcons, and many other predatory birds might appear threatening, reflecting insecurity—although eagles can also represent power and pride. Song birds can suggest inspiration, hope, a fresh start. The owl is traditionally a creature of wisdom and insight. The magpie, a thieving bird, may hint that someone is robbing you of something— perhaps contentment or potential. If the bird is injured in your dream, you may need to nurture yourself back to well-being in some way, or possibly there are flaws in a relationship. If you're the bird, perhaps there's a situation you're trying to fly away from.

FLOWERS

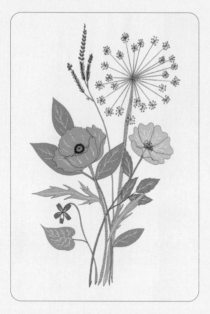

If flowers manifest in a dream, they are typically a symbol of comfort, beauty, kindness, love, or joy. They may represent your capacity for faith or compassion. Color symbolism may operate: white denotes purity; blue, calm; purple, adventure; pink, tenderness; orange, creativity; and yellow, playfulness. The type of flower can be significant, too, so it's worth researching traditional associations. Daisies may suggest friendship; roses, love; dandelions, childhood; and lilies, endings. The condition of the flowers may be a message from your dreaming mind about your inner life. Are they wild, cut, garden, or artificial flowers? Are they fresh and blooming or wilting and dying? If you receive a bunch of flowers or are picking them, this suggests a promising new relationship may be on the horizon. If you see a flower growing in a desert or barren soil, this may be a reminder of your resilience—your ability to overcome challenges.

INSECTS/REPTILES

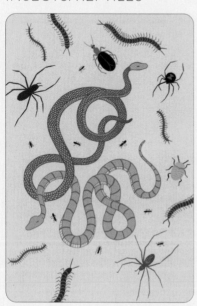

Within the animal kingdom, reptiles and insects carry a strong symbolic charge with largely negative overtones. In dreams they typically represent worries or threats in your waking life. A reptile can indicate emotional coldness or possibly a situation or relationship you would benefit from dealing with rationally rather than emotionally. A snake, traditionally symbolic of deviousness, could be a sign that greater honesty is required, either from you yourself or from someone you're involved with. Insects tend to represent irritating problems or distractions. A spider may symbolize a small issue that could become larger if attention isn't paid to it. However, spiders can also denote patience, or the success attainable through skill and hard work. If any creature in a dream takes monstrous form, with exaggerated size or features, this is probably about coming to terms with your shadow side, or aspects of yourself you find hard to accept.

TREES/MOUNTAINS/GARDENS

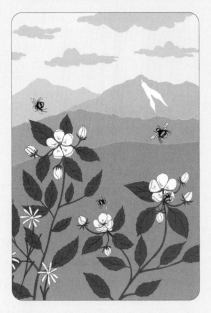

Because they are landscape features, trees in a dream may seem incidental, but they often refer to your spiritual and emotional development. Forests typically symbolize the unknown. They may reflect feelings of being lost or confused. If so, the way out is to trust your intuition: such a dream gives a clear sign you need to find inner strength and reconnect with what truly matters. The denser and gloomier the wood, the more urgently you need to move towards clarity and contentment. However, if the mood is of wonder or joy, the dream may point to the benefits of deeply exploring the mysteries of the self or of life itself. A mountain indicates a challenge you must overcome: the view of the valley below is the reward for persistence. Gardens refer to areas of potential growth in your life. Grass suggests a desire to be closer to nature or to your natural self.

WATER

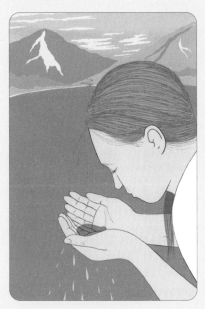

Water is a symbol of your emotional state, with associations of change and flow. If you're going through a tough time emotionally, a water dream may suggest you'll pass into a new phase. Whatever form water takes (rain, snow, river, lake, waterfall, sea), it's also a symbol of refreshment, healing, or new beginnings. This is so even if you dream of a storm, since all weather is temporary. If water in a river or lake is clear, this is a sign of emotional honesty and resilience; if it's dirty or muddy, this indicates insecurity and perhaps overreliance on support from others. A swimming pool is a symbol of emotional restraint. A shower or bath suggests you need to cleanse yourself of negativity. Swimming reflects a positive attitude if you're moving through the water happily; but if you're struggling or going against the current, or getting submerged, your emotions may be overwhelming you.

BODY PARTS

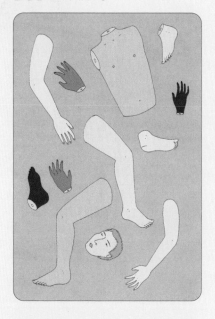

Body parts represent aspects of your personal identity and the clue to their meaning lies in the associations you have with the specific body part. For example, if you dream of arms this could represent your ability to reach out to others. Hands suggest attention to detail, whereas legs indicate your ability to move forward; feet are your foundation or what keeps you grounded. Heads represent your intellect and necks are the connection between your physical body and your mind. Blood is a symbol of your essence or life energy and muscles are your strength. Hearts point to your relationships and bones your support system. If a body part is injured something is preventing you from expressing the quality represented by that specific body part. If you dream of teeth, skin, hair, nails, or other body parts that you shed this suggests the need to let go and move on from a situation or mindset that is holding you back.

BOOKS/WRITING/WORDS

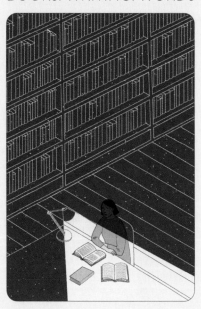

Books in a dream may symbolize a search for knowledge. If lots of books appear, perhaps you're letting details obscure the bigger picture or being abstract or theoretical when you'd do better to be practical. If you're reading a book, you may be on a quest for personal development. If the subject of a book is apparent, it's likely to be significant, as a warning or encouragement related to that theme—for example, a travel guide could reflect an urge to see more of the world or to get away from home, or a fear of losing your way. If you're searching for a book, this can indicate overreliance on others' opinions. If you're writing, or writing materials are apparent, again the dream may be urging you to come to your own conclusions. Specific words written down or in print usually require self-analysis before the meaning dawns on you: look out for ambiguities.

CELL PHONES

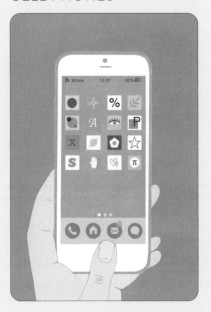

A phone represents your ability to communicate. So if in a dream you're having technical problems with your phone, or are unable to get a signal, or you've left it at home or lost it, perhaps you're unable for some reason to get your message across in waking life. Alternatively, there might be someone who isn't being clear—be sure to bear in mind the possibility that this person is you: perhaps you need to be more honest or direct. If a text or email appears in your dream, this may be a symbol of fast communication: your unconscious may be urging you to move forward without delay on a project or resolution of some kind. Dreams about texting may also indicate a need or desire to be more direct—or conversely an anxiety that plain speaking runs the risk of revealing some uncomfortable truths.

CLOTHES

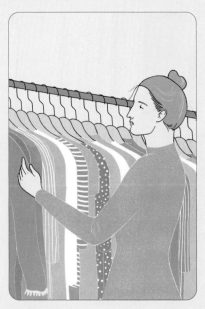

The clothes you wear in a dream may indicate the image others have of you. If there are clothes in a wardrobe or lying around, the reference may be to how you'd like to appear. The color and condition of the clothes are significant. If they are gray and threadbare, you may be lacking in self-esteem or feel you aren't realizing your full potential. Brightly colored or designer items may indicate you feel on top of things—or would like to be. If you're wearing the wrong outfit, that's a sign you have problems accepting who you are. Wearing someone else's clothes suggests there's something about that person you admire or can learn from. Putting on clothes suggests moving forward hopefully. Undressing indicates shedding inhibitions or outmoded beliefs or habits. Hats represent aspirations; shoes, what is keeping you grounded; and jewelry, the qualities you most value in yourself and others. All three occur commonly in dreams.

FOOD OR DRINK

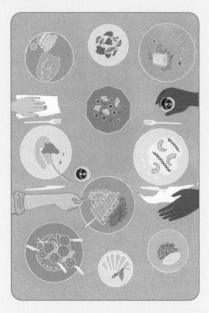

Food or drink tends to refer to emotional, spiritual, or intellectual nourishment. It represents qualities you're seeking or need to seek for your personal development. Hunger or thirst suggests that you're striving toward wholeness or contentment or possibly neglecting basic needs. More particularly, hunger may indicate a need for greater material security or emotional or sexual fulfillment; thirst can suggest a longing for deeper meaning. Occasionally what you're consuming will be significant—eggs might suggest a new start, milk a return to childlike dependency. Eating alone could suggest independence or loneliness, depending on your circumstances. Overeating suggests self-indulgence. Drinking alcohol may indicate you're trying to suppress difficult feelings, but it can also mean a desire for more stimulation. If you dream of eating glass, or some other dangerous substance, you or someone in your life could be struggling to deal with (swallow) a painful situation.

MONEY

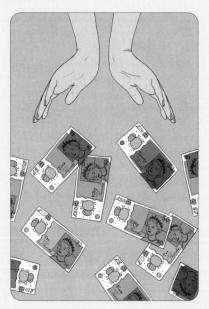

Money in a dream (appearing as cash or credit cards) can be a symbol of how emotionally secure you feel. It can also represent the influence you feel you have over others. Any dream featuring a bank, investment, money transfer, or will can similarly carry an emotional meaning. Giving money away or spending suggests a wish to be more generous or outgoing; alternatively, your unconscious may be urging you to be more giving in a relationship. Receiving money indicates you need to accept or ask for emotional support. If you find money, whether by chance or after searching for it, there's something valuable about yourself you need to learn—perhaps you're already close to discovery. Losing money symbolizes a lost opportunity. If money is stolen, you may believe you don't deserve something or someone in your life, or that others are taking you for granted.

MUSICAL INSTRUMENTS

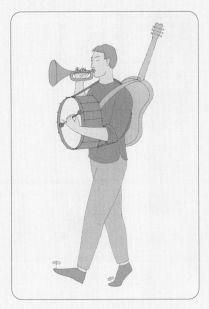

Anything to do with music in a dream generally has positive associations. Music evokes emotion, so to hear it in a dream connects you with the flow of your inner life. Of course, if the music is dissonant, your attention is being drawn to emotional discord; a beautiful melody suggests the opposite. If you dream of performing music, the instrument may be significant. The black-and-white keys of a piano suggest seeing things clearly, or perhaps a need for you to find harmony between two extremes. A violin may be a call for a gentler approach, although it can also suggest you need to pay greater attention to details. Playing percussion may be a sign that you need to drum up more support or that something needs to be drummed into you. Singing in a dream is a symbol of joyful self-expression and may reflect a desire to be more creative.

NUMBERS

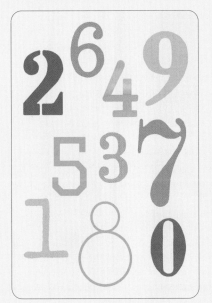

Numbers in a dream can be significant. Some initial possibilities to consider are: house or apartment numbers, phone numbers, and meaningful dates (for example, birthdays or anniversaries). A dream about your own PIN may suggest you're being too secretive or self-centered. If a two-digit (or more) number fails to reveal meaning, try looking at the individual digits in turn. If you're still stumped, take a numerological approach: numerology looks at the symbolic meanings of numbers, especially in terms of spiritual growth. In brief, number 1 suggests new beginnings; 2, relationships; 3, creativity; 4, stability; 5, change; 6, nurturing; 7, truth; 8, wealth; 9, awareness; 0, timelessness and eternity. In general, odd numbers are perceived as possibly anxious or threatening, and even numbers as more reassuring and positive. Of course, small numbers can appear as things. If, for example, there are two horses in a dream, perhaps they represent a significant pairing in your life.

SHOPPING

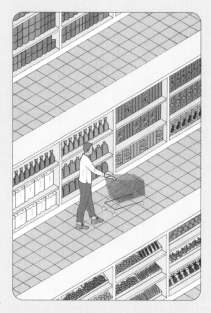

Stores in a dream can indicate what you want or think you need in life to be happy. Also, shopping represents choice: the possibilities on offer, the decisions you need to make, the attitudes or responses available to you. Browsing in a shopping mall, department store, or market, or window-shopping downtown, may be a prompt for you to review your opportunities. The particular items on sale may narrow down the dream's meaning. If you're buying clothes, you're seeking protection but also an identity. If it's food or drink, you need to attend to your basic emotional needs. If you can't find the item you're looking for, this is a sign of some general frustration with life, or of a particular need or desire that isn't being satisfied. If you're shoplifting, a part of you may feel the only way to get what you want may be to break the rules.

SOCIAL MEDIA

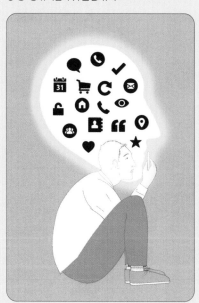

Online communication is an inescapable part of modern life, so it isn't surprising that many of us dream about Facebook, Instagram, YouTube, or the like, or communicating via messenger apps. In general, these kinds of dreams suggest a desire to expand your online network or to either reconnect with people from your past or seek out new horizons. If you dream of changing your profile photo or page, this indicates that you want to control the way other people see you—or may already be doing so. If you find yourself scrolling aimlessly or being directed to the same web page repeatedly, perhaps you're spending too much time online. Gaining likes or new online followers may reflect a feeling that you're worthy of others' approval, whereas losing friends or followers may indicate that you can't or won't conform to the expectations placed upon you by friends, family, or society.

TECHNOLOGY

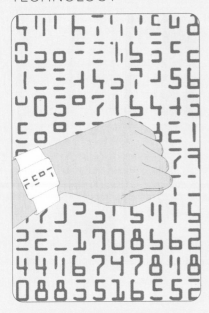

Computers, laptops, and tablets occur very commonly in dreams; so do heavier pieces of hardware such as elevators or escalators. Often the technology malfunctions or proves frustrating in some other way. If it's a computer, your files may get deleted or corrupted, or you're unable to access them or receive messages or emails; if it's an elevator, the mechanism sticks. We think of technology as a servant programmed to obey our bidding. Hence, devices that malfunction in a dream show that we aren't in as much control of a situation or relationship as we think. In your interpretation consider the purpose of the technology. A dysfunctional email system may imply that you're struggling to connect or communicate your true feelings to someone, or being insufficiently clear or emphatic about your needs. If this doesn't fit, look for other sources of frustration the dream may reflect—something obstructing your career? The feeling that technology is passing you by?

TRANSPORT

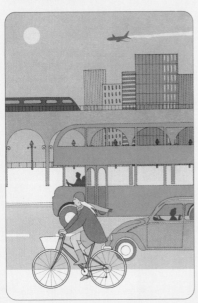

Any mode of travel is likely to convey a message about the way you're making progress in your life. The most significant question is whether or not you're driving (or navigating) or are just a passenger—the latter scenario suggests you're being passive and might benefit from taking more control: you need to drive your own life forward. The direction and speed of travel will offer further interpretive clues. Aircraft in dreams suggest new experiences and excitement. Bicycles indicate a need for balance: there may be opposing forces (or people) you need to reconcile. If you're in a bus or coach, this suggests conformity. Given the associations water carries, boats or ships point to an exploration of your emotional life. Trains can mean you're too dependent on others, or insufficiently flexible, though if you're the driver perhaps others depend on you. Cars represent the image you present. Caravans or trailers can suggest an unconventional approach.

ACTOR/CELEBRITY

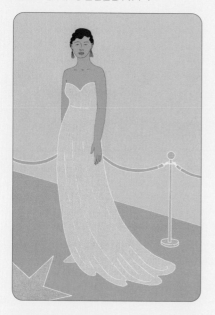

When a celebrity or actor (or even a historical figure) appears in a dream, the significance may lie in what they are famous for, their personality, or behavior, or the way they project themselves to others. The person may represent some aspect of yourself you need to acknowledge or integrate, or a quality you seek to emulate. Consider what the person represents to you. If they are an actor, perhaps it's a role they played that speaks to you? If you dream you're a celebrity, or are intimate with someone famous, this may indicate your desire for greater attention and/or success. If you appear in a TV show or movie in a dream, perhaps you feel you're playing a part in waking life. Appearing as the star may be a warning against self-importance; conversely, being a supporting actor may mean you should put yourself center-stage more.

BABY/BIRTH

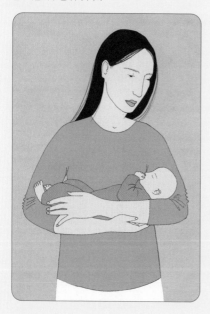

If a baby appears in a dream, or you give birth, this is an indication of new beginnings or creativity within yourself. Since a baby can't survive unless taken care of, the dream may be encouraging you to give more support or attention to someone or something. The baby's behavior could be significant. If they are content, you might be adequately nurturing your inner gifts; if they are distressed, you're perhaps being neglectful. Sometimes a dream about a baby or pregnancy can be simple wish-fulfillment. However, if this is inappropriate to your circumstances, it could also be an attempt by your unconscious to help you reconnect with your inner child or discover your hidden potential. If a baby is born with an adult head, this may point to intellectual maturity combined with emotional naïveté. Pregnancy dreams often indicate a period of waiting during which you need to be patient.

CHILDREN

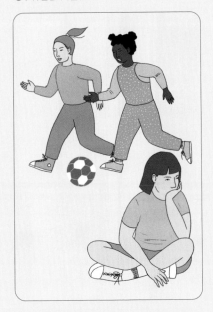

Children in dreams tend to be positive signs, symbolizing joy, spontaneity, or warmth. Depending on your circumstances, they could also indicate a desire for more fun, energy, or innocence. Another possible interpretation is that a dream child represents your attitude to your own childhood. The meaning could also relate to any current feelings of vulnerability or dependency you may have. Forgetting or losing a child is a reminder to focus your energies in waking life on what truly matters. Perhaps you're focused more on providing for your family than on being with them? This is a common issue in the work/life balance dilemma. Dreams of unborn children you may one day have suggest future potential you have yet to identify or focus on. In rare instances such dreams may indeed show your unconscious mind crossing the boundaries of time and space to glimpse your future intuitively.

DECEASED PEOPLE

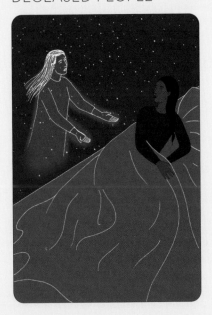

There's a spiritually minded school of thought that sees dreams of departed loved ones as genuine signs of the afterlife—a way for the deceased to gently reassure you that they are eternally alive in spirit. Research shows that in 85 percent of cases people who have afterlife dreams feel better able to cope with their grief. Regardless of your beliefs, dreaming about a lost loved one can be comforting if they passed away less than two years ago. If, however, it's longer than that, perhaps you've not yet fully processed your grief. Dreaming about the dead could denote they still have a strong influence over you. If a ghost or spirit appears, this could symbolize unfinished business. It may also represent lack of clarity in your thinking or in some situation you're dealing with. Alternatively, something or someone is haunting you— perhaps an old lover or a regret.

ELDERLY PEOPLE

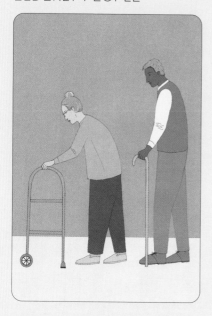

Dreams that feature anyone old sometimes signify lessons the past can teach you, though at the more obvious level they may relate to worries about our aged loved ones becoming frail and/or dependent or about our own prospects as we endure the aging process. If we find an old face troubling, perhaps the dream is trying to tell us that we should be more accepting; after all, with age comes wisdom. Consider how the old person in the dream shows their age: if the face isn't visible, perhaps it's through reduced mobility or old-fashioned clothes. Either of these aspects may be key to the dream's meaning: are you perhaps worrying that you can no longer keep up with fashion, or is your freedom of movement limited by factors beyond your control? If you or someone else ages suddenly in a dream, this could reflect a deep-seated wish to halt time.

FAMILY

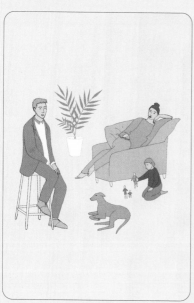

If you dream of a family member, this might be related to issues between you. However, there might be a less direct meaning. If you dream of your father and he's a figure of authority for you, this might suggest you need to bring more discipline into your life. If you dream about your mother and she's a nurturing person, maybe you need to take better care of yourself. If your brother or sister is outgoing and you're introverted, a dream about them could suggest you aspire to their qualities. Every family member can represent an aspect of your own personality. If you dream of family members arguing, this might reflect tensions within your own psychological make-up. Recurring dreams about parents might suggest you need to be more independent of them. Dreams of children often reflect fears about their safety or success or the possibility they are moving away from you.

PEOPLE

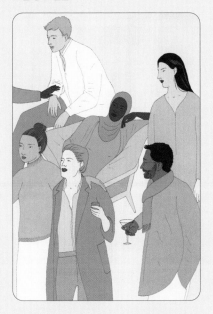

Frequently, people in a dream will represent aspects of your own personality or preoccupations. This is true of friends and acquaintances, but it can also apply to strangers—useful to remember when you have a puzzling dream about someone you've never met. The key to understanding might be what they say or do, rather than who they are. People working together might suggest the importance of cooperation—perhaps you envy a relationship that seems more harmonious than your own, or perhaps you feel isolated in your job and would like more contact with others. People bumping into each other may denote frustration about individuals who are involving themselves in your personal affairs, or simply a deep-seated wish for more solitude. If people are present when you are doing something private (such as using the bathroom), this usually indicates insecurity or low self-esteem.

RELIGIOUS OR SPIRITUAL FIGURES

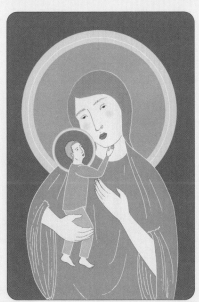

A spiritual leader (such as Jesus, the Buddha, or Muhammad, or an anonymous priest or nun) or a religious symbol (such as an angel, cross, star, or crescent moon) probably indicates moral or spiritual issues in your life. You're being urged to find a way forward. The dream is unlikely to be directing you toward a particular faith or belief system. More probably it represents your desire for guidance, comfort, or support. There may be an emptiness you seek to fill, or a sense of confusion, a craving for a moral compass. Perhaps you'd benefit from a role model on life's path. There are important decisions to be made, and you'd do well to seek guidance from either your best, most insightful self or from some external source of wisdom. You need to take your focus away from material concerns and place it on higher values—the things that truly matter in your life.

SEX

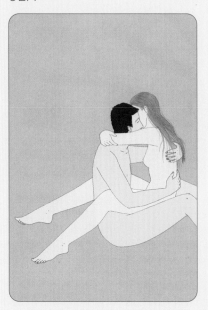

Dreams about sex aren't really about the physical act. They are more about your desire for greater connection and intimacy. This may include a craving for more physical closeness, but the main emphasis is likely to be emotional. Such dreams may also suggest the need for psychological growth and self-discovery. Perhaps it would be helpful to deal with hidden or conflicting aspects of yourself. The identity of your sex partner in the dream is crucial to the meaning, since they will represent aspects of yourself you need to open up or integrate. You don't actually want to sleep with them—there may just be something about them you admire or can learn from. Or if you find this person repulsive, perhaps you must acknowledge or address a part of yourself you find uncomfortable. Anything associated with sex in a dream may also indicate hunger for greater excitement or adventure, or just trying new things.

WEDDING/MARRIAGE

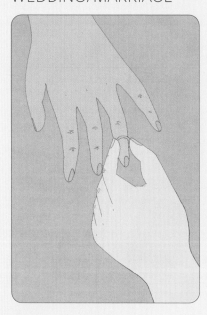

Dreams that feature a wedding or marriage are usually all about new beginnings—often with no literal reference to married life. This interpretation applies to all wedding-related details—bride, groom, bridesmaids, usher, wedding cake, ring, proposal, and so on. Such symbols indicate the potential for moving from one phase of life to another with excitement, commitment, and love. Most often such dreams will refer to relationships, but they can also point to a leap forward in your professional life or, more generally, your personal development. At a deep psychological level, a marriage may represent the masculine and feminine aspects of yourself (animus and anima) uniting, or a balance of reason and emotion. If you're the bride or groom in a dream, pay close attention to the person you're marrying, as their character may suggest what aspects of yourself you need to learn from or assimilate to become whole.

BEACH

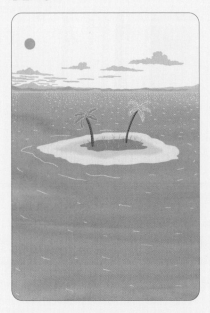

A sandy beach on a tropical island indicates a longing to escape your everyday routine and responsibilities—this is a common wish-fulfillment dream. Beaches are places where water (emotion) meets earth (the body), so such a dream could also suggest a longing to express your emotions—that is, enact them bodily. Do you stay on the beach in your dream or take a swim in the ocean? The answer could affect the meaning. If there are footprints in the sand, this could indicate something from your past you're moving away from, since eventually those footprints will be washed away. If the sand shifts under your feet, maybe you're concerned that your life lacks stable foundations. If the dream emphasizes the island itself, or you're alone on the beach, this might suggest feelings of isolation or insecurity, or else a need for some time alone to reflect on what really matters.

BUILDINGS

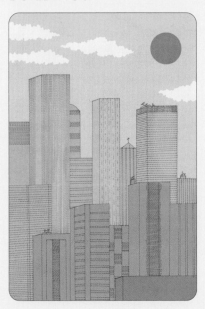

Buildings tend to represent your sense of self. Pay attention to what kind of building it is. If it's your home or a house, this suggests that your personal life is your paramount concern at the moment; if it's an office or factory, professional life may be your preoccupation. If you're inside, are you on the ground floor, upstairs, or in the basement? Generally, the main floor represents the present moment, the lower floors your shadow aspects, and the upper floors your higher self. Being outside the building may convey a feeling of being detached. Any doors in your dream could suggest opportunities, while windows could represent your openness to new ideas. Any stairs may be a comment on how you feel about your social status, or else they could refer to a period of transition. The ceiling represents what you may feel is limiting your progress.

CASTLES/ANCIENT BUILDINGS/TOMBS

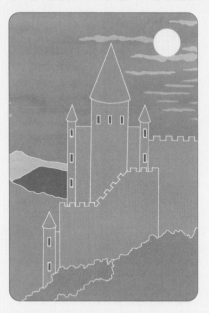

A castle, like a house, can be interpreted as the ego or your inner world. However, castles were built specifically to protect. Seeing one in a dream suggests you need to put up barriers—perhaps someone or something has the potential to overwhelm you? Perhaps you've built your defences already—if so, are they protecting or imprisoning you? Any other impregnable building—even a bank or government building—can have similar associations. With any ancient structure perhaps there's a reference to time. Your dreaming mind could be urging you to look to the past for inspiration or guidance. Any kind of tomb or memorial might suggest that someone who has died or belongs to your past can inspire you; or you might have buried a part of yourself that you need to either bring back to life or leave behind and mourn. You may also need to resolve your feelings about the inevitability of death.

SCHOOL

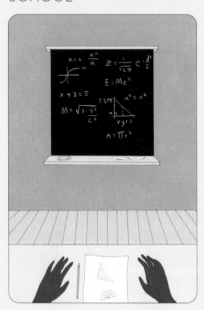

Dreams of being a pupil at a school or some other place of learning usually relate to lessons you need to learn in your waking life—perhaps a basic principle or skill you've forgotten. There may be an opportunity to learn something new that you've either missed or need to pay more attention to. Have you learned from past mistakes or are you repeating them over and over? If you're a child in the dream, this might suggest that you need to bring some childlike simplicity to a current situation: complications in your waking life may not be as difficult as they seem. If you're a teacher, mentor, or lecturer, the message of the dream could be that you need to be your own guide and inspiration. Perhaps the answers you're seeking can't be found by asking other people: true guidance must come from within.

UNFAMILIAR, SECRET, OR UNUSED ROOM

TOP 10 DREAM

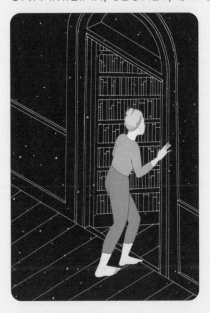

A house or home in a dream is a symbol of yourself. As with you, there'll be an outside and an inside. The rooms in a dream house symbolize aspects of who you are on the inside. Therefore, rooms that are unknown, locked, or secret indicate possible areas of personal transformation that are not yet being expressed—either you aren't aware of them or for some reason you aren't capitalizing on them. The key to interpretation is what was in the room, as this may give you an indication about an aspect of yourself that is undeveloped or undiscovered. If the room is empty or deserted, this suggests you aren't taking steps to get to know your own strengths and talents: inspiration is waiting to happen. Bear in mind that a hidden room can also be where your dark side is to be found: you need to face this aspect of yourself and come to terms with it.

WORK

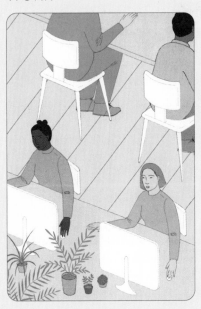

Not surprisingly, since most of us spend so much time working, dreams about work are common. If the dream features a job that isn't yours, it isn't urging you to make a career change. Instead, it's using symbolism to highlight a characteristic you need to integrate into your personality. Being a writer may suggest you need to extend your communication skills, being a teacher that you aren't explaining matters well enough to others. If the dream is about your job or workplace, it will often focus on what you find unsatisfactory—or what you'd change if you had sufficient self-knowledge to identify the problem. If you're performing a mindless task or being overwhelmed with a giant in tray, you may feel you're losing identity at work—you might need to assert your needs more. If you're on a treadmill, this could relate to a nonwork context, even to a relationship.

FINDING SOMETHING VALUABLE

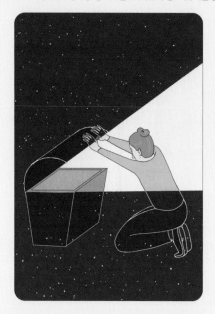

Discovering something valuable—a hoard of antiquities, hidden treasure, or just modern banknotes—suggests that in waking life you might be on course to learn something important about yourself or about a situation or relationship. Finding something beautiful can have the same meaning, even if the value isn't apparent. Consider the object's symbolic associations—if it's jewelry, that could indicate that you're looking for a way to present yourself more confidently and attractively; if it's something historic, that could mean you're learning from the past. If what you've found is mysterious (for example, an instrument whose purpose you don't know), you may need some radical change that will make life clearer. Other people finding something valuable suggests you may need to reach out to others and ask for help. If you give a found object away to someone else, maybe you aren't valuing your own talents enough.

FLYING WITHOUT WINGS

TOP 10 DREAM

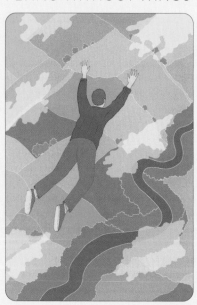

Flying without wings in a dream is almost always an exhilarating, positive symbol. It's a celebration of something happening in your waking life that gives you (or will soon give you) a high. Perhaps you feel you've achieved, or are on the brink of, something significant. This deep satisfaction can relate to relationships, travel, your professional life, or a personal project (whether creative or practical in nature). However, it may also come from a sense of freedom, the lifting of restrictions after a period of confinement, or perhaps a leap forward in your personal development.

If the flying is easeful, this confirms the idea that you're feeling self-assured and positive— euphoric even. Pay attention to the direction you're flying in: upwards, or flying high, suggests spiritual growth or worldly ambition; downwards, or flying low to the ground, suggests newfound determination and strength; backwards suggests happy memories.

MOVING FORWARD

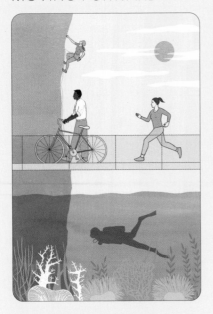

Walking in a dream, like any other form of travel, is a symbol of the discoveries you're making as you move forward in life. It's generally a positive dream, because you're relying on your own resources to get where you need to be. The surroundings, and any obstacles or diversions you encounter, will give you a clue about your progress. If you're walking in mud, there may be a messy situation in your personal life. Walking on glass suggests you're feeling hurt. Being barefoot may indicate a need to be more authentic. Moving on air suggests self-confidence and positivity—though there may be risks involved and possibly a certain amount of bluffing. Climbing (or hiking in rugged terrain) suggests challenges you need to overcome. Walking indicates you're judging the pace of change well—as opposed to running, which may suggest an impatience to reach your goals.

SUPERHERO POWERS

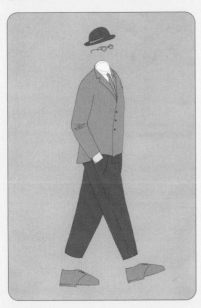

Dreams in which you have superhero or magical powers are typical of childhood, but you can have them at any age. Perhaps you're faced with malevolent forces but discover you have supernatural abilities to resolve the conflict—whether strength, flight, telepathy, X-ray vision, or clairvoyance. Generally, such a dream suggests that you're tackling some kind of problem in waking life and would prefer it if the issue just magically disappeared. However, an alternative is that there's some hidden talent or potential within yourself you need to discover and develop. Being invisible may seem like a superpower but it can also be a sign you feel ignored or neglected in waking life, or feel your life is insignificant to others: the dream is urging you to be more assertive or self-motivated. The opponent in a superhero dream may be a rival in love or work, or perhaps an aspect of yourself.

Text by Theresa Cheung

Theresa Cheung has a degree from King's College, Cambridge, and has been researching and writing about spirituality and personal transformation for over 20 years. She has two *Sunday Times* top 10 bestsellers to her credit and her numerous bestselling titles include *The A to Z Dream Dictionary* (2019) and *21 Rituals To Change Your Life* (2017). Her books have been translated into over 40 different languages and her writing has been featured in national newspapers and magazines. Media appearances include a debate about spirituality with Piers Morgan on GMTV and Russell Brand's *Under the Skin*.

Illustrations by Harriet Lee-Merrion

Harriet Lee-Merrion is an award-winning illustrator based in Bristol, UK. Her work has appeared in publications including the *New York Times*, the *Washington Post*, and the *Guardian*, and has been exhibited in New York, London, and Berlin.

LAURENCE KING

Laurence King Publishing Ltd.
361–373 City Road
London EC1V 1LR
United Kingdom
www.laurenceking.com

Magma for Laurence King

Text © 2019 Theresa Cheung
Illustrations © 2019 Harriet Lee-Merrion
© 2020 Laurence King Publishing Ltd.

ISBN: 978-1-78627-706-0

Text by Theresa Cheung
Illustrations by Harriet Lee-Merrion
Design by Mylène Mozas

The Dictionary of Dreams text has previously appeared in *Dream Decoder*, published by Laurence King Publishing Ltd. in 2019.

Printed in China

Laurence King Publishing is commited to ethical and sustainable book production. We are proud participants in The Book Chain Project ®
bookchainproject.com